COMPUTERS IN MEDICINE

BY EVE AND ALBERT STWERTKA

A COMPUTER APPLICATIONS BOOK
FRANKLIN WATTS ■ 1984
NEW YORK ■ LONDON ■ TORONTO ■ SYDNEY

Allen County Public Library
Ft. Wayne, Indiana

Photographs courtesy of:
AP/Wide World: pp. 2 , 50, 72;
University Hospital, State University of New York at
Stony Brook: pp. 11, 15, 59; The Methodist Hospital: p. 32;
Brookhaven National Laboratory: pp. 44, 45;
Kurzweil Computer Products: p. 77; James Prince: p. 86.

Library of Congress Cataloging in Publication Data

Stwertka, Eve.
Computers in medicine.

(A Computer applications book)
Includes index.
Summary: Describes the many ways computers are used in the medical field, such as in diagnosing disease, admitting hospital patients, and helping the handicapped to read, talk, and hear.
1. Medicine—Data processing—Juvenile literature.
2. Medical Care—Data processing—Juvenile literature.
[1. Medicine—Data processing. 2. Medical care—Data processing] I. Stwertka, Albert. II. Title. III. Series.
R858.S79 1984   610'.28'54   84-7249
ISBN 0-531-04846-2

Copyright © 1984 by Eve and Albert Stwertka
All rights reserved
Printed in the United States of America
5 4 3 2 1

YOUNG ADULTS
STO

ACPL ITEM
DISCARDED

Y 610.285 ST9C
STWERTKA, EVE.   2253503
COMPUTERS

Y 610.285 ST9C   2253503
STWERTKA, EVE.
COMPUTERS IN MEDICINE

ALLEN COUNTY PUBLIC LIBRARY

FORT WAYNE, INDIANA 46802

You may return this book to any agency, branch,
or bookmobile of the Allen County Public Library.

DEMCO

CONTENTS

CHAPTER 1
New Circuits to Health Care
1

CHAPTER 2
A Computerized Hospital
10

CHAPTER 3
The Central Computer and How it Works
20

CHAPTER 4
Body Imaging
30

CHAPTER 5
More Tools for Diagnosis
47

CHAPTER 6
Intensive Care
56

CHAPTER 7
Research Through
Data Banks and
Computer Modeling
64

CHAPTER 8
Computers to Aid
the Handicapped
76

Index
89

COMPUTERS IN MEDICINE

The authors are most grateful to the following individuals
and organizations whose help made this book possible.

At North Shore University Hospital, Manhasset, New York, to:
Bob Brody, Department of Biostatistics
Stanley Gross, M.D., Department of Laboratories
Roger Hyman, M.D., Department of Radiology
John Morrison, M.D., Cardiopulmonary Division
Peter Reiser, M.D., Department of Medicine
each of whom contributed a great deal of precious time
and invaluable expertise to our enterprise. Our gratitude,
also, to Karen Dech and the staff of the Department of
Community Relations, who arranged all our meetings.

At Stony Brook University Hospital, Setauket, New York, to:
Dennis Gai, Manager of Computer Systems Development, whose
lucid presentation and tour of the facilities allowed us
insight into the workings of a fully computerized hospital.

At Long Island Jewish/Hillside Hospital,
New Hyde Park, New York, to:
James Moyer, Director of Management Information Systems,
who kindly gave us an introduction to his field.

CHAPTER 1

NEW CIRCUITS TO HEALTH CARE

The time may not be far off when patients going to see a doctor will start out by telling their symptoms to a computer. Sitting in front of the keyboard, they will push buttons to answer questions appearing on a video screen. "Hello, Mrs. Colby!" the computer might reply after the patient has identified herself. "Have you come for your yearly checkup? (Press Y to answer Yes, N to answer No) . . . Are you currently experiencing a health problem? (Press Y or N.)"

Computer interviewing is already being used by a few hospital admitting departments. Experience has shown that in mental health clinics, for example, some people feel more comfortable, at least at first, using a keyboard and video screen than talking about their problems to a human professional. In addition, there are many routine questions to be asked of every patient before the doctor can diagnose the illness or recommend the proper treatment. Such

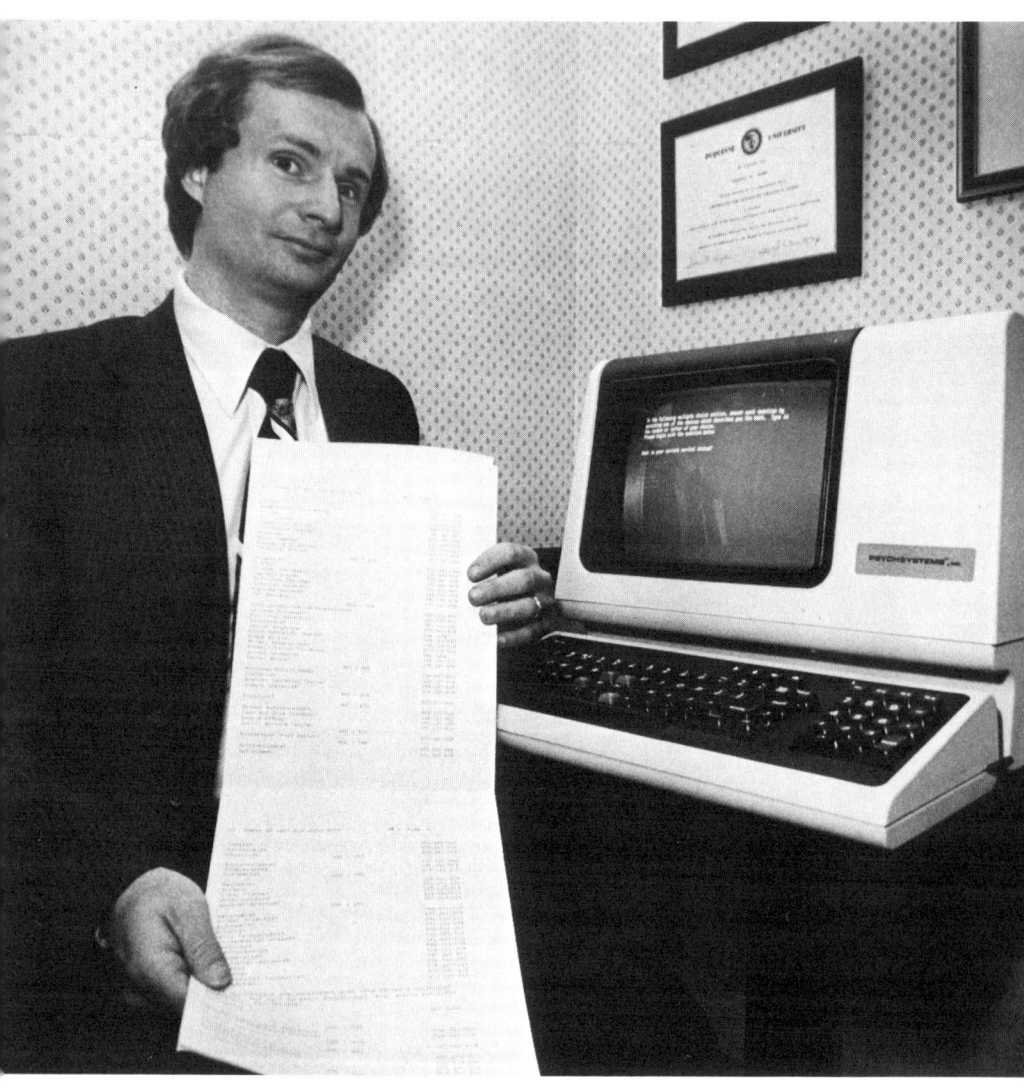

Dr. Terrence DeMay, a Pittsburgh psychologist, is shown here with the test results from a computer that administers standard psychological tests to new patients with mental health problems.

questions take much of the doctor's time. Using a computer to take care of the preliminaries leaves the doctor more time for talking to patients.

A computer interview does not involve asking all patients exactly the same questions. Built into the interview program are the possibilities of branching off in different directions. Each new question asked by the computer depends on the patient's answer to the previous question. From the main stem, or trunk, of the interview, lines branch off in different directions. Experts use the word "decision tree" to describe a computer program structured in this treelike way. The first point of branching, for example, might come at the question "Are you male or female?" Depending on the answer, the program would proceed along two slightly different lines of questioning. Later in the interview, the program would again branch off to special sets of questions for patients answering yes to questions such as "Do you smoke cigarettes?" or "Have you ever had a heart attack?"

In fact, the very first words to appear on the screen might be a list of languages from which patients can choose the one they best understand. For those who pick *español,* for example, the entire interview would then continue in Spanish. Other patients might choose to be interviewed in English, Korean, or any other language included in the program.

When the interview is completed, the patient may be given some medical tests. The doctor's technical assistants then add the results of any laboratory tests or X-rays to the computer questionnaire. By the time patient and doctor sit face to face, a complete printout of interview and test results lies on the doctor's desk. Results can also be scanned on a desktop video screen. And, for the doctor's use, the computer has translated the layperson's language used by the patient into medical terminology, which is a mixture of Latin and English.

COMPUTERS AS DECISION MAKERS

From interviewing patients by computer, it is just a few steps to computerized diagnosis and suggested therapy. Some people are uneasy at the idea of a computer taking over the doctor's role of diagnosing illness. Others point out the computer's advantages. For one thing, the computer has a perfect memory, while even the best doctor cannot possibly memorize or recall at will all the data needed in medicine today.

Computer programs that diagnose and recommend treatment already exist in many medical specialties. Often, they are used for teaching in medical schools. Students can test their own diagnostic skills against those of the program. Diagnosis by computer also acts as a sort of physician's consultant in hospitals and doctors' offices. One such program was prepared by a kidney specialist, Dr. Howard Bleich of Harvard University. Dr. Bleich's program examines the test results of each patient's metabolic functions—the sum total of the body's physical and chemical processes. Because these processes interact in complicated ways, the data is very numerous and time-consuming to analyze. In spite of this complexity, the computer takes only seconds to produce a list of probable diagnoses. Not only that, it explains the reasoning behind its conclusions, suggests suitable treatments, and warns of possible complications to watch out for. Sometimes, it asks for more information. It always ends by recommending articles in recent medical journals to help the doctor update his knowledge.

Dr. Bleich defends the computer's role in diagnosis. For one thing, he says, it never gets tired or careless. "It works day and night, weekends and holidays, without coffee breaks, overtime, fringe benefits, or human courtesy." Sometimes, Bleich feels, it even outperforms him. After all, he worked on the program in stages, only when his ability to concentrate was high, and had the help of many brilliant colleagues.

In remote places, access to a medical computer program saves lives. In such places, a small staff often has to cope with a great variety of health problems. A computer can act as a lifeline to the latest findings and recommended procedures. In this way, sick people in outlying areas can get up-to-date diagnosis and treatment.

One day, medical computer programs may even make house calls. Through cable TV, a subscriber could use a tone-coded dial, instructing a central computer to communicate with him via his own TV set.

With all their intelligence, computers are unlikely to become robot substitutes for human physicians. Even very complex programs are still limited and inflexible compared to the human intellect. Still, in the last few years, computers have transformed the way many physicians do their work.

We will begin, here, by introducing two very different examples of computer use in medicine. Then, in the following chapters, we will report in greater detail on the work of computers in hospitals and in the medical community as a whole.

COMPUTERIZED ORGAN BANKS

In the spring of 1983, a young woman suffering from an acute, fatal liver disorder was lying in the University of Pittsburgh hospital. Doctors knew that only the implant of a new liver from a donor in good health could save her life. Day after precious day passed, however, without turning up a suitable donor.

Then, in early June, an eighteen-year-old Californian was killed in an automobile accident. Raymond Camacho had been driving home from a birthday party held for him by his friends when his car struck a tree. At the hospital, he was pronounced brain-dead even though doctors managed to keep his vital organs functioning on a life-support system. In their grief, his parents decided to give some measure of life to their son by donating his organs to science. Part of him would live on by giving life to others. Raymond's liver was sent to Pittsburgh University Hospital, where surgeons performed the long operation of implanting it in the young female patient. Raymond's heart and one kidney went to the Medical College of the University of Virginia. Patients in Raymond's native Miami received his eyes, skin, thigh bone, knee joint, shoulder, arm, and other kidney. Altogether, more than sixteen people received transplants from Raymond Camacho.

The hospital in Miami where Raymond died and the hospitals in the other states where the organs were sent all belonged to a computerized organ registry. An organ registry is a central information source that medical workers in any participating hospital or surgeon's office can search at any time simply by pressing a few computer keys.

Computers also play another vital role in organ donation. Although transplants save many lives, they are still surrounded by problems. The cell-tissue types of both donor and recipient must be very similar. If they do not match, the recipient's body soon rejects the donated organ. Organ compatibility depends on substances called antigens found in the walls of the body's cells. A person's particular antigens are thought to be determined by heredity. If the donor organ carries antigens not present in the recipient, the latter's immune system manufactures defensive antibodies and eventually rejects the donated part.

With the help of computers, doctors are now making safer and more permanent transplants. The process that prepares a recipient for organ transfer is called tissue-typing. Laboratory workers examine the tissue cell of tens of thousands of subjects each year to see what antigens they carry. More than thirty major antigens have to be identified and matched. All thirty antigens must match; a single foreign antigen could trigger a rejection response.

The larger the pool of both recipients and donors, the better the chance of finding a suitable match. But the job of tissue-typing would be terribly time-consuming without a computer to analyze and store the wealth of information.

Speed, of course, is essential in organ transplants. If the donor is deceased, the organ must not be allowed to deteriorate. Computerized tissue-typing is done in minutes. A hospital staff member then transfers the data to a national organ registry, informing the medical community that particular organs of a certain tissue type are available. The computer also searches its waiting list of patients to come up with the names of closely matching recipients, the hospitals where they are waiting, and the doctor in charge of each case.

COMPUTERS IN SPECIAL SURGERY

When Lois Eaton was born, her parents were concerned about the strange shape of her head and face. They consulted Dr. Jeffrey Marsh of the Washington University Medical Center in St. Louis, a specialist in corrective surgery of the skull.

One of the problems of corrective surgery is that doctors often cannot foresee the exact kind of malformation they will encounter when they operate. X rays alone do not give enough information. To wait until the actual incisions are made means making on-the-spot decisions; this is not always the best way to proceed.

To enable him to plan his operation with care, Dr. Marsh and his team took a series of painless computerized tomography (CT) scans of Lois's head. In CT scanning, the computer divides the imaged body part into numerous cross-sections, very much like the stacked slices in a loaf of bread. In this case, there were thirty-nine cross-sections. Using diagrams obtained by computer graphics, Dr. Marsh's team actually made lucite models of each section and assembled them into a life-size replica of the child's head. (You will learn more about CT scanning and computer graphics in Chapters 4 and 7 of this book.)

After reviewing all the computer data, the team of doctors were able to see clearly what had happened. The left side of Lois's skull had grown normally, but the bony plates on the right side had fused too early and prevented normal growth.

With the help of an expert in biomedical computing, Dr. Marsh devised a model of the right side of Lois's head, symmetrically matched to the left side. One week before he operated, he was able to show this model to Lois's parents on the computer screen. What he had learned allowed him to plan the operation with care. He knew exactly where he would need to loosen the frontal plates to allow growth, where he would have to use bone graft, and what sort of mold he would have to cast for an artificial implant. The computerized images allowed him to see even soft tissue, such as muscle and fat, instead of only bone.

The Eatons were delighted with the results of Lois's surgery. As soon as the child was brought out of the operating room her parents could see that her head was now normal in shape and size and that she was a very pretty baby.

The technique used at Washington University Medical Center employs a combination of many skills. Its three-dimensional computer graphics were originally developed for the design of automobiles and airplanes. Dr. Marsh worked with a computer graphics expert and an aircraft design engineer at nearby McDonnell Douglas to adapt the graphics for his purposes. Sophisticated computers at McDonnell digitize the scans made of a patient's skull. (To digitize means to translate sensory data into numerical values.) Then, the same program that designs the structure of an airplane wing converts the data into a "wire frame" computer image. This image, which looks like a three-dimensional head modeled of thin wires, can be manipulated on the computer screen. The viewer can actually rotate it, or view it from above or below, inside or outside. Different mathematical values are assigned to the various kinds of tissue. These are shown on the screen in degrees of brightness or in contrasting colors so that viewers can distinguish between muscle, fat, and bone. The program also allows the viewer to "strip" away parts of the structure or to superimpose images of one part on another.

New research will use the computer to predict growth patterns, not only of bone but also of soft tissue. This is a very important consideration in operating on children. The improvements made by surgery have to take into consideration that a young patient's tissues will grow and change considerably for many years to come.

CHAPTER 2

A COMPUTERIZED HOSPITAL

One of the first hospitals planned from the start around a central computerized information system was Stony Brook University Hospital in New York State. When Stony Brook opened its doors in 1980, its user-friendly, interactive, real-time computer was ready, too. These terms mean that most people can use the system easily, without the intermediary help of a technician, that it can be hooked up to exchange information with other machines, and that it processes information immediately instead of in batches, as older systems do. It is on the job around the clock, every day of the year.

DATA INPUT

About 140 terminals and about half as many printers are located all around the hospital. At every nursing station, you can see a terminal keyboard, a video screen consisting of a cathode ray tube (CRT), and a printer. In addition,

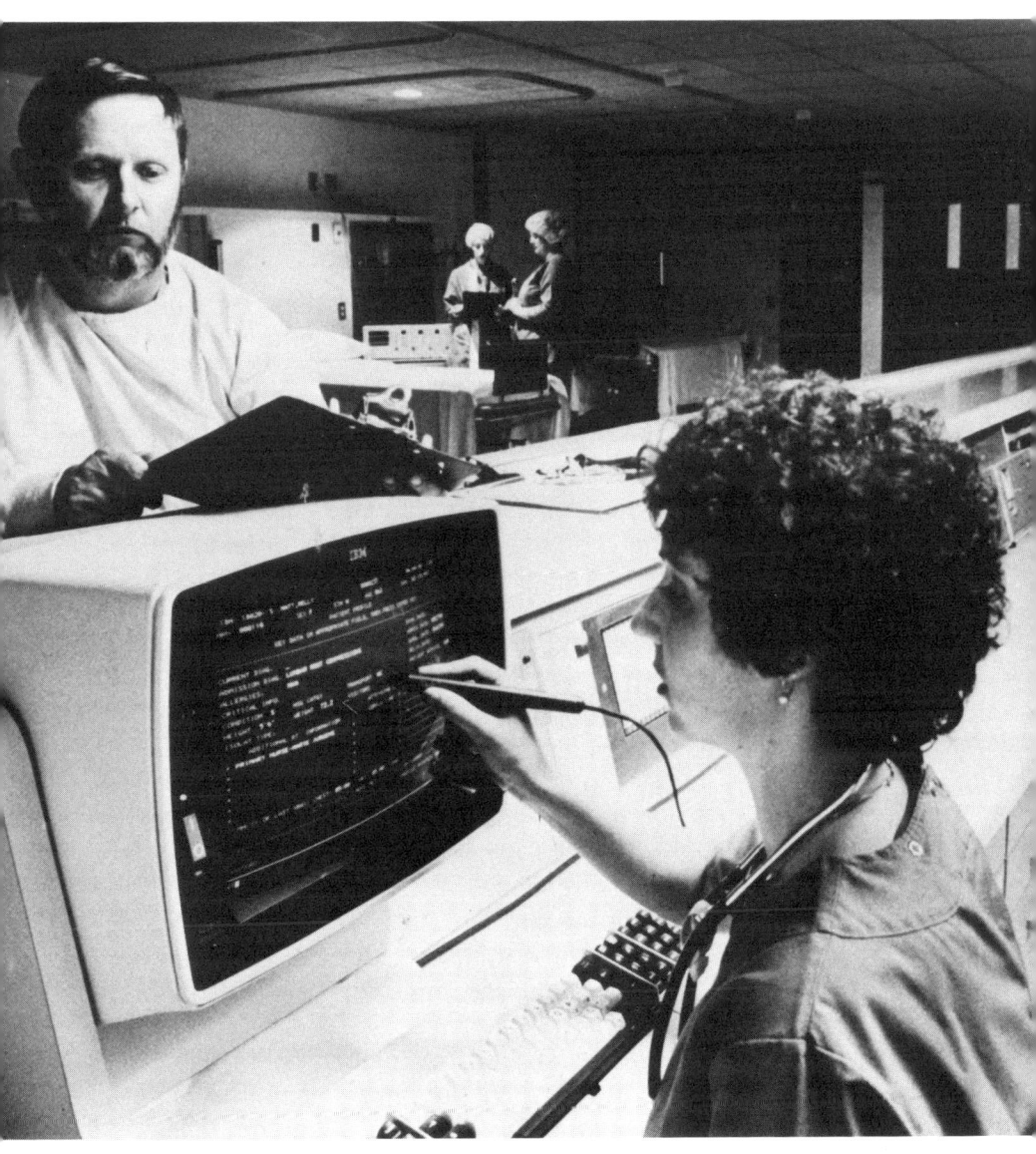

Patient information, following surgery, is entered into the computer with a light pen at one of Stony Brook University Hospital's many terminals.

mimicomputers dedicated to special purposes are used in nearly every department. The chemistry laboratories, for example, use many different automated analyzers. Test results are collected right from these instruments through cords that run to an IBM Series I minicomputer that collects the results—each labeled with a patient identification number—and sends them on to the hospital's central data base. A surgeon in the operating room who needs the immediate results of his or her patient's blood test, only has to look at the CRT screen next to the operating table to find the information.

Three different methods may be used to enter data into the system. First, hospital staff members can type it on the keyboard. Many standard items of information come ready-made, in the form of "canned" texts in the computer's memory. These items can be entered or retrieved by pressing a single code key. In fact, about sixty percent of the information on patients' records is prerecorded.

A light pen, which looks like a long, thin flashlight, is another instrument for talking to a computer. "Is the patient allergic to penicillin?" appears on the CRT screen, followed by "Yes" and "No." Pressing the tip of the light pen to the correct answer and flicking a tiny switch activates the system. The CRT senses the light, and the computer accepts the information.

The third way of feeding in data is directly from the hospital's many different instruments. Among these are devices that analyze blood and that monitor a patient's heartbeat.

Information can also be drawn out of the system, using the keyboard and the light pen. Suppose a doctor quickly wants to scan the intermediate results of a test that takes several steps to complete. He or she can call them up and read them off the screen. Later, when a paper copy of the complete test is needed, the computer can be instructed to type one out on the printer.

WELCOME TO ADMITTING

Which beds are occupied and which ones are empty? Who are the patients in the hospital at any given moment, and where are they? Most hospitals can't answer these questions exactly. But those with computerized systems always have an up-to-the-minute census on hand. The computer keeps track of patients as they are moved to the X-ray department or the operating room or simply to a bed with a brighter view. Admitting clerks know from moment to moment which beds are about to become free.

A large hospital receives hundreds of calls daily from doctors or surgeons requesting beds for their patients. If you were sitting before the computer at the admissions desk, trying to locate a bed for a patient named Rupert O. Brown, you would first of all want to know if Brown had ever been a patient at your hospital before. To do this you would press the Patient Identification Inquiry key. An alphabetical list of patients appears on the screen. Among the many Browns who are listed, you notice: Brown, Rupert O. His sex is indicated M for male, and his birthdate matches that of the patient you are trying to place. Mr. Brown has been here before. With a touch of the light pen to the name, Brown's previous admission record appears on the screen. Most of the needed information is already there, including the type of insurance he carries and whether he came in previously as an emergency patient, an outpatient, or an inpatient. Now, when Rupert Brown comes to the hospital to be admitted, you need only to update the information already in the computer.

Mr. Brown's symptom is chest pain, and he is being admitted for coronary bypass surgery. The logical place to find him a bed is the cardiac unit of the hospital. You press the Bed Census key on the terminal. The list appears on the screen in front of you. You scan the rooms on the cardiac floor and see that bed 542A is unoccupied.

Next, it is your job to inform the floor nurse that the

new patient is on his way up. You touch the necessary keys. At the nursing station on Floor Five, the electronic printer begins its quick rat-a-tat. A nurse leans over and tears off the printed message. And even before Rupert Brown has stepped out of the elevator, his completed admission form is in the nurse's hands. At the same time, a notice has automatically reached the housekeeping department that bed 542A is now occupied and will need a daily supply of sheets and towels.

Before Brown can undergo surgery, his doctors need to know the exact state of his health. This will be determined by means of a full set of tests. While Brown undresses and climbs into bed, the nurse recalls his admission record on the CRT screen and enters more information. Is the patient allergic to penicillin? Is he currently taking medication? The answers to these very important questions must be on file.

Now for the tests. The nurse touches the key for Order Entry. A form appears on which dozens of different routine tests are listed. Such a listing is often referred to as the "menu." The nurse orders from this menu all the required laboratory tests and X rays Brown will need. The nurse does this very quickly by touching the end of the light pen to each line on which a needed test is listed. The computer notifies a technician, who comes to take samples of blood. At the same time, the computer alerts the lab that blood samples are coming and tells Radiology that a patient is about to arrive for X rays. As Rupert Brown is wheeled down the hall, the nurse informs the computer that the patient is in transit to the Radiology unit.

After surgery, Brown will be moved into the cardiac Intensive Care Unit, where a special minicomputer will watch over his vital signs and record them. When he recovers sufficiently and moves back into the regular part of the hospital, his vital data will not be lost. The minicomputer interfaces with the mainframe computer of the hospital so that his record will always be kept up-to-date.

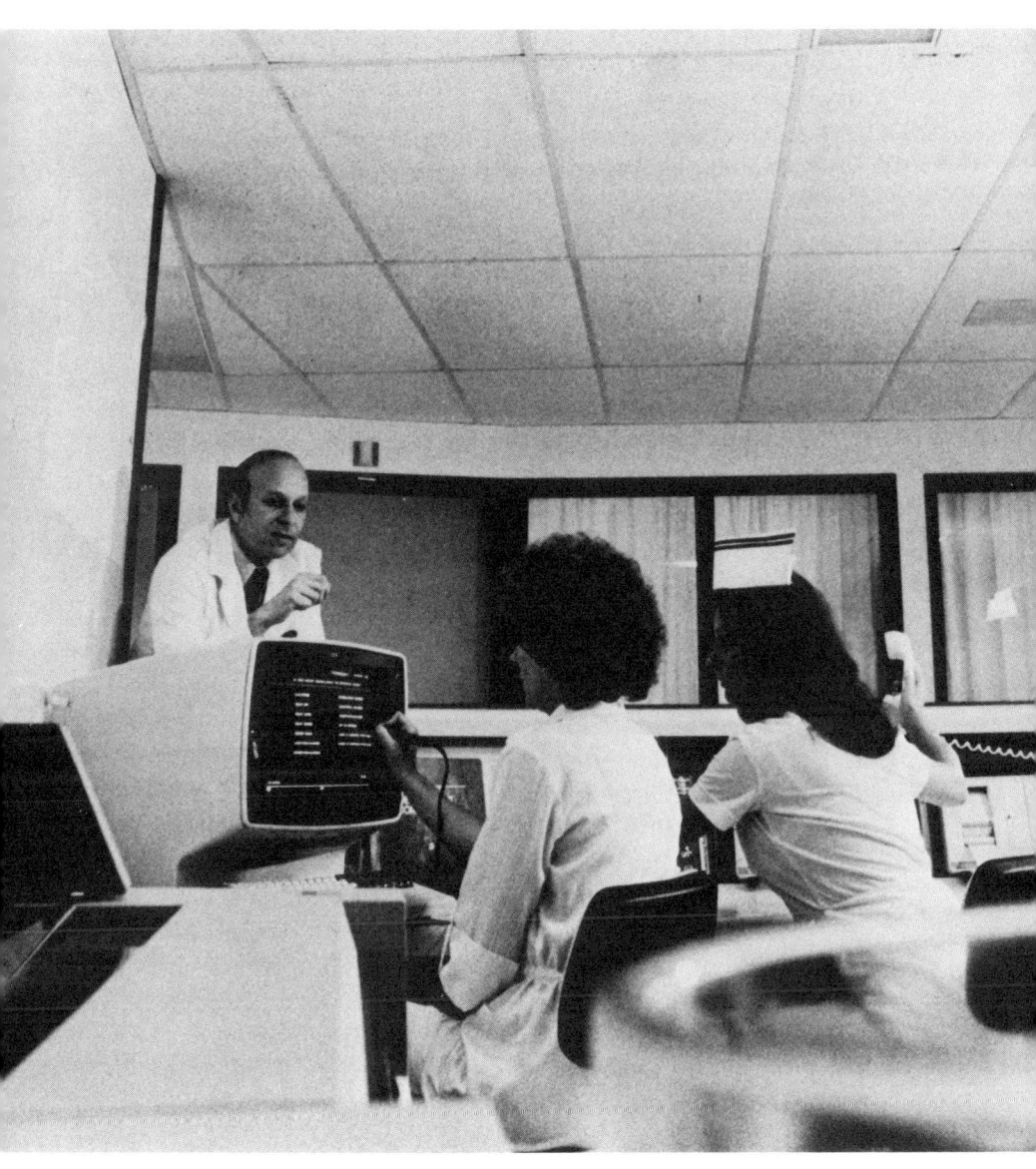

Doctors can order laboratory and radiology tests from computer terminals in the patient care units of Stony Brook University Hospital.

As floor nurses and doctors order each procedure during a patient's hospital stay, the computer captures this information for yet another purpose, the so-called back end of the entire process. Under headings such as Laboratory, Pharmacy, Anesthesia, Operating Room, Therapy, and TV Rental, the computer lists and adds the charge for every service. When Rupert Brown has recovered from his operation and is ready to be discharged from the hospital, his bill will be ready, too, and will be handed to him straight from the printer terminal.

When patients are discharged, they often need instructions for further home care. This may include dressings for wounds, baby-feeding formulas, special diets, or physical therapy. The computer is then used to print personal directions, complete with emergency telephone numbers and a list of scheduled checkup appointments.

SPECIAL FUNCTIONS

A computer system such as the one we are describing can be programmed to perform so many useful services, large and small, that it is impossible to mention them all. For example, it can display conversion tables for various measurements, or drug compatibility charts listing combinations of pharmaceutical drugs that are acceptable and others that are harmful or even lethal. It can indicate what legal steps must be followed in admitting a "dangerous" mental patient. (How is "dangerous" legally defined? The computer will tell you.) It can give its users access to outside data banks and services such as MED-LINE, a constantly updated medical information system. It can also function as an electronic mail service, whereby people all around the hospital can send each other instant keyboard-to-printer messages. In fact, the same message can be sent to any number of printers at once: to all nursing stations, for example, to the operating rooms, or to three or four staff members who are needed at a meeting.

The computer can be programmed to display data in innumerable patterns for special uses. If the director of laboratories wants to know which were the most frequently ordered lab tests during any given day, month, or year, the computer can tell him this.

Every hospital collects data on the kinds of diagnoses, treatments, and procedures it provides. An international code (the ICD-9 code) is used to unify these studies, which tens of thousands of hospitals participate in all over the world. Among other things, the data serves to determine whether an institution offers primary, secondary, or tertiary care. Primary care describes the kind of care given in a doctor's office or at a small clinic. Secondary care describes the treatment obtainable at an average community hospital. Tertiary care is the most sophisticated in terms of both technical equipment and expertise. It is available chiefly at teaching hospitals.

Together with the institutional cost report—also prepared by computer—hospitals use these figures to set their fees. Or rather, since the cost of treating a patient always exceeds the charge, hospitals use these figures to negotiate the amount of money insurance companies will pay to reimburse patients for treatment at a particular institution.

KEEPING THINGS CONFIDENTIAL

In a large hospital, some eight hundred people are likely to have access to the central computer. Indeed, it would be an invasion of privacy if all eight hundred freely read everything about each patient's condition. To prevent this, terminal stations are programmed to recall only the amount and kind of information needed for a particular job. At the visitors' center, for example, the only things the receptionist can find out from the terminal screen is whether a certain patient is in the hospital and where he or she is located. In areas where more detailed information can be obtained, personnel must use a password and an identification code to get access to the computer.

Only certain supervisory offices are equipped with a "master screen." From here, a complete electronic survey of the hospital is possible. For instance, a touch of the keyboard will reveal the present status of the Emergency Room, showing how many patients are there and what is wrong with them. Similarly, one can call up the chemistry laboratories' worklist to see which tests were completed that day and which remain to be done.

From the master screen, one can even find out how many employees happen to be using the computer keys at any given moment. This helps the hospital determine the peak hours of computer use. At those times, responses from the computer come back far more slowly than during the hours when demand is low.

SAFETY

The most widely used hospital information system was formulated by Duke University and developed commercially by IBM. An institution such as Stony Brook University Hospital can impose its own character on this basic structure, transform it, and branch out into new areas. To do so, the institution uses a test system, separate from but, at the outset, identical with the main one. The two systems run side by side, but changes and innovations are developed on the test system to make sure it works correctly. In a hospital, patient safety always comes first.

Occasionally, the main computer must be shut down for repairs. When this happens, an announcement is broadcast over the public address system to warn everyone that the computer will be down for a certain length of time. Then, routine work, such as admitting and bookkeeping simply stops for a while. Of course, intensive care units, surgery, and other critical areas have their own independent minicomputers. When the main computer is down, these areas keep on functioning, using records stored on tapes or disks. If one of these minicomputers fails, an emergency alarm sounds, and a substitute computer, kept ready on a crash cart, is quickly wheeled into its place.

Should the main computer be down for more than an hour or two, a backup paper-handling system goes into effect. Paper forms for such an emergency are kept under all desks. When the paper system is in use, some of the employees are pressed into service as messengers, running back and forth with lab reports and interoffice mail in the old-fashioned way.

As a further safety measure, each terminal in the hospital carries a REPAIR key, to alert a service crew whenever the terminal is not functioning properly. For example, the screen might be dim, response time might be unusually slow, or the printer might be stuck. Pressing the REPAIR key not only puts in an automatic service call, it also calls to the screen a checklist of common problems. By picking the item that most closely applies and touching it with a light pen, the operator informs the repair crew of what needs to be fixed.

But, you might ask, what if some disaster happened to the main computer? What if earthquake, flood, or fire engulfed the entire computer area? Would all that stored-up information be lost forever?

To prevent the calamity of losing patient records and research data painstakingly collected over many years, the hospital maintains a complete duplicate set of records in an offsite storage area. The location is far away, and its whereabouts are kept confidential.

CHAPTER 3

THE CENTRAL COMPUTER AND HOW IT WORKS

In the basement of the hospital, visitors come upon a large, cool, gently humming room. This is the domain of the computers. Very few human workers are seen here. It is as though the machines ran things all alone. In fact, up to a point, they do.

Here stands the main computer—a tall presence in blue and white metal. Magnetic disks are spinning inside the computer's translucent plastic frame. Hundreds of such disks are ranged in a storage area on one side of the room. Other computer consoles of various sizes stand all around. Each has a somewhat different function.

Most computerized hospitals handle data by the so-called distributed processing method. A central database is used, but there are also numerous stand-alone units, usually mini- or microcomputers. Stand-alone units gather their own information but are capable of "handshaking," or communicating with, the mainframe computer.

Some hospitals also buy service from a data-handling company that specializes in adding up and sending out bills. When doctors and nurses order services on the computer terminal screen for a patient, the information is called up for billing purposes by the main computer. The main computer forwards this data through a telephone wire to the billing company, which may be in a distant city. Because this company handles bills for hundreds of organizations, it is very efficient and saves the hospital some of the expense of this time-consuming chore. This procedure is called a turnkey operation because the customer need only turn a key or a switch to have the service performed.

THE CENTRAL PROCESSING UNIT (CPU)

The central processing unit (CPU) controls the entire computer system. Like the human brain, it has a memory and the ability to perform logical and arithmetic operations. The CPU must take the programs written in English by the technical staff and translate these detailed instructions into a "machine" language understood by the computer. Following these instructions step by step, the CPU performs all the necessary calculations. Using the data fed into it from terminals at other locations, the processor must then present the results of its analysis in a form that will be most useful to doctors and hospital personnel.

A basic computer system, of course, consists of several other important units of "hardware." There are the nput devices that make data available to the processor unit, and the output devices on which the results of the processing are displayed. There are auxiliary storage debices and "network" controllers. Along with all the remote terminal data stations, there is also a console terminal.

The CPU must synchronize all of these units. The faster it can communicate with its own internal units, such as memory and control, the more effective it will be in coordinating remote stations. The faster it can take in, or "access," data and execute instructions, the more useful it will be in solving complicated problems and quickly producing useful output.

The heart of the CPU is a clock that controls and coordinates all the functions of the CPU. In the form of a oscillator, the clock beats at a steady frequency and makes sure that all the electrical impulses within the CPU are properly sequenced. The greater the frequency, the faster the CPU can operate. The CPU of the IBM 3031, for example, has a 6 megaherz clock (six million cycles per second). In other words, its clock beats at the incredible rate of six million times every second. This permits the CPU to handle large quantities of information both quickly and efficiently.

THE COMPUTER CONSOLE

In the computer room, an operator communicates with the central processor through the console terminal. Flashing lights, dials, and buttons found on the computer console serve to inform the computer operator of exactly what the processor is doing at any given time. The console terminal consists of a typewriterlike keyboard and a cathode ray tube (CRT). While the computer is running, it is constantly sending messages to the operator, regarding different operations and needs. For example, the system may write a message on the CRT, indicating that there is some malfunction in part of the system or that paper is required in the printer. The operator can also use the console to question the computer system, say, to determine which tasks are currently being carried out and which will be carried out next.

BITS AND BYTES

Some eleven thousand transactions run through the central computer per hour. In more technical terms, this translates into five billion bytes, or five gigabytes.

Unlike human beings, who have learned to think and count in the decimal system, computers do their arithmetic in a system that counts only up to the number two. In a modern computer, almost all calculations are done in this base-two arithmetic, and data is stored in the form of units called "bits" (*B*inary dig*its*). A bit can assume only one of two possible values. It can be thought of as being either "on" or "off," or if numbers are assigned, as being either zero (0) or one (1).

The computer can sense whether a bit is "on" or "off" by using special electronic components built into its hardware. Some older computers make this determination by using a small ring-shaped piece of material called a magnetic core, which can be magnetized in one of two directions. Most computer systems today use a semiconductor memory, where the status of a bit is indicated by whether or not electricity is flowing along a circuit. Semiconductor storage has greatly increased the speed with which data can be accessed by the processor. The time needed to access data stored in a semiconductor is measured in nanoseconds (billionths of a second), some ten times faster than in a magnetic core.

The actual data in computer storage is represented by a series of eight bits called a "byte." Similar to a code, a given combination of bits, consisting of any number of either "on" or "off" units, defines the value of a byte. In one commonly used coding scheme, the Extended Binary Coded Interchange Code (EBCDIC), a byte consisting of a given sequence of eight bits is assigned to every number, to every letter of the alphabet, and to special symbols such as punctuation marks. When a character (the number, letter, or symbol) is read into the computer's memory, it is stored there in a byte of storage.

NETWORK CONTROL

With billions of bits flowing hourly in and out of the computer in all directions, you may well wonder how the traffic is controlled. It is all done by an ingenious machine called the communications or network controller, which acts as an electronic traffic cop for the entire system.

The communications control unit is the main link between the computer room and the outside. A wire goes into it from the computer, and a tree structure of communication telephone lines goes out from it to other data-gathering stations. It routes all the messages to and from the computer. (The advantage of remote terminals is that they permit many users to "timeshare" the tremendous computational power of the central mainframe.)

Contact between a remote terminal and the central computer is usually established by the network control unit "polling" each terminal linked to the system. It asks if there is any data to send to the computer. If the answer is no, the next terminal on the line is asked. When the computer sends data to a terminal, a technique called "addressing" is used. Special signals are generated by the communications control so that a particular message will be sent to the right terminal, or "address." When computers communicate with each other, they need to make sure they are speaking the same language. A "line protocol" translates between computers. The communications protocol is a set of "handshaking" rules that accomplishes the movement of data from one machine to another.

MODEMS

Communication lines are generally standard telephone lines, and a telephone system, of course, is designed to carry sound. But computers speak to each other in a silent language of electronic impulses, with pairs of impulses representing bits, not sound. Remote terminals, therefore, cannot be directly connected to these lines.

To allow data in the form of bits to be transmitted over telephone wires, it must first be converted into sound impulses. This transformation is performed by a device called a modem (derived from modulator-demodulator). A modem can also reverse the process and change audible tones into digital signals. Both the sending and the receiving end of the communication line require a modem, so a system with thirty-two remote-control units will require thirty-two modems. After the modem has done its job, the communications control, if it is receiving data from a remote terminal, can assemble the transmitted "bits" of information and send them on to the main computer for further processing.

AUXILIARY SYSTEMS

Not all the information received by the computer is intended for immediate use. Pharmacy medication records, admission and discharge records, blood donor-recipient records, to cite but a few examples, must somehow be stored for future reference and yet not take up precious space in the internal memory of the computer. Since the main memory of most computer systems is not large enough to contain all the programs and records kept by the hospital, a secondary storage system is required. Much of the data gathered by the computer is stored in this auxiliary system. The two most commonly used auxiliary storage devices are magnetic tape and magnetic disks.

MAGNETIC TAPE

Magnetic tape, similar to the tape found in an ordinary audio cassette recorder, is made of a plastic material called Mylar. The tape is coated with iron oxide so that it can be magnetized. The length of tape on a reel can be as much as a half mile (2,400 feet, or 720 m) long. Computer operators mount these reels on high-speed tape drives so that data can be quickly read from or written onto the tapes.

Data is stored on the tape by a computer-controlled electromagnet that produces magnetic spots on the tape to represent binary digits. Arranged in vertical columns across the width of the tape, the spots are capable of "writing" more than 6,000 bytes per inch (2.5 cm).

Reading from the tape is just the reverse of writing. The tape is placed over a "read head," where an electrical impulse is produced in the electromagnet whenever a magnetized spot appears. Data can be transferred from the tape to the main computer at rates as high as 1,200,000 characters per second.

Tape is somewhat inefficient for storing certain types of records because it stores data in a "sequential" manner—one record after the other. This means that access to a particular record requires each record on the tape to be read in turn until the desired one is found.

MAGNETIC DISK

Magnetic disks are circular metal platters some 14 inches (36 cm) in diameter that resemble blank phonograph records. Both surfaces are coated with a metal oxide so that data can be magnetically stored. These disks are typically assembled into packs of eleven platters, all mounted on a common hub with a half-inch space between disks. A pack is capable of storing two hundred million characters of data. Computer operators can easily mount these packs—or remove them—from disk drives.

A spindle in the disk drive unit will rotate the disk pack at a constant speed of approximately 3,600 revolutions per minute. Data is recorded on the disks by means of arms inserted into the spaces between the disks. The arms contain an "actuator" electromagnet that floats above the surface of the disk and produces magnetic spots that correspond to the bits of data being recorded. When reading, the actuator senses the spots on the surface and transfers the data to the computer.

As the disk is spinning, the data is recorded in the form of concentric circles called "tracks." The number of tracks on a disk can range from 250 to over 800 per recording. Of great importance is the fact that the actuator can be positioned over one of the tracks in less than 50 milliseconds (1/20th of a second). This means that direct, or so-called "random" access, to stored information is possible without first going through an entire sequence of other records. The obvious advantage of random access is speed. When an inquiry is made regarding a certain patient, the computer randomly accesses the records for the name or number and retrieves the information without having to read any of the other records first.

DATABASES

Hospitals organize much of their stored information so that it can be easily accessed by researchers and doctors. Often, medical records are used in more than one program. It would be inefficient and wasteful to store the same data in many different locations. Collections of data from various sources are, therefore, made available throughout the hospital out of a single special storage unit called a database. The database, an important component of the "software" configuration of the computer, contains a collection of data that is independent of the programs using it. If one wanted to know the location of a certain patient, for example, one could find that out from any terminal in the hospital.

The database administrator at the hospital, often called the DBA, investigates what information is needed most frequently and establishes the database. It is also the job of the DBA to make sure that the security of certain types of information is not violated, since access to data stored in a database can be controlled at one central point.

SAFEGUARDING THE SYSTEM

The "nerve bundles" of the computer brain are its wires and cables. There are thousands of these, kept safely out of sight and away from traffic. Lift up one of the large square floor panels of the computer room and you will uncover a space of about 3 feet (.9 m) deep that runs under the entire floor on which you are standing. Here you will see the network of cables, neatly laid out in thick, black or colored strands.

Although a great deal of power surges through the wires, the room is always cool. Air conditioning keeps it at approximately 70°F (21°C) even in summer. Above 80°F (27°C), delicate electronic equipment no longer functions properly. Its precision-tuned parts must not be subjected to the expansion and contraction ordinary materials undergo with great changes in temperature.

The hospital buys its electricity from the local power company. To be on the safe side, the cables leading into the building run underground. Even so, the people who planned the central computer room had to reckon with a possible power failure. They placed emergency lights on every wall. If a power failure occurs, these lights take over. Emergency diesel and gas turbine generators go into action, and ten seconds after the blackout, twenty-five percent of the hospital's power supply can be restored. This is enough to keep the main computer running.

Fire, of course, is one of the greatest dangers in any electrical installation. The best way to put out electrical fires is to deprive them of oxygen. Releasing carbon monoxide into the area would smother the fire, but it would also kill any persons who happened to be in the room.

Instead, the system uses halon, a purple gas that is not lethal to humans. It is stored in a pressure tank outside the building. If smoke or heat tripped the alarm system, halon gas would come pouring into the computer room through ports in the walls, both above the floor and in the cable region below.

There is only one thing wrong with halon: it is very expensive. So, whenever staff members run a fire drill, they release only a small amount of halon—just enough to make sure everything is in working order.

REPAIRS AND EMERGENCIES

What happens when the computer goes out of order? A typical hospital buys its repair service from a large company, such as IBM. But the shortest response time one can buy is two hours, and in a medical emergency every minute counts. This is why several minicomputers on crash carts stand along one wall of the central computer room. These carts are ready to be wheeled to any site in the hospital within four minutes.

CHAPTER 4

BODY IMAGING

The ability to see inside the human body has always been one of the primary goals of physicians. Until quite recently, though, they had to depend on their sense of touch, exploratory surgery, or conventional X-rays to get information about the inside of a patient's body. These procedures were either limited in their usefulness or invasive and possibly damaging. Today, however, the computer's ability to absorb vast quantities of data and make rapid calculations has led to the development of several new ways to image the internal organs without surgical intervention.

COMPUTED TOMOGRAPHY

The development of computed tomography (CT) precipitated a revolution in the field of medical diagnosis. Consisting essentially of combinations of X-ray devices and computers, the CT scanner has become one of the most powerful diagnostic tools in medicine. It allows doctors to clearly photograph the body's soft tissue and targeted internal organs. Most major hospitals now have access to CT scanners, and more than one million patients receive scans on these machines every year.

A major shortcoming of conventional X-ray analysis is that structures in front of, or behind, the particular part being investigated appear on the film and are sometimes difficult to distinguish from the targeted organ or region. Instead of trying to compress a three-dimensional structure into a two-dimensional picture, computed tomography produces an image of only a thin slice (*tomos* in Greek) of the body. This slice is usually taken at right angles to the long axis of the body, which explains the original name, computed *axial* tomography, or CAT. Many individual slices can be taken and put together like slices of bread that form a loaf.

The image produced in computed tomography is formed by combining a large number of X-ray absorption measurements made through the chosen slice at different angles. The information from all these scans is then given to a computer, which generates the final image. The mathematical technique used by the computer is largely the work of Allan McLeod Cormack and Godfrey N. Hounsfield, for which they were awarded the Nobel Prize for Physiology and Medicine in 1979.

In a modern CT scanner, the patient is made to lie on a table that is motor driven to get the patient inside a large doughnut assembly called a gantry. A laser alignment system that illuminates and outlines exactly what cross-section of the patient's body is to be examined is used for accurate positioning of the body.

The gantry contains a rotating X-ray tube and approximately one thousand solid-state detectors on a stationary ring. As the X-ray tube rotates about the patient, it can produce more than a thousand views, each a different angular projection of the patient. Each view results in

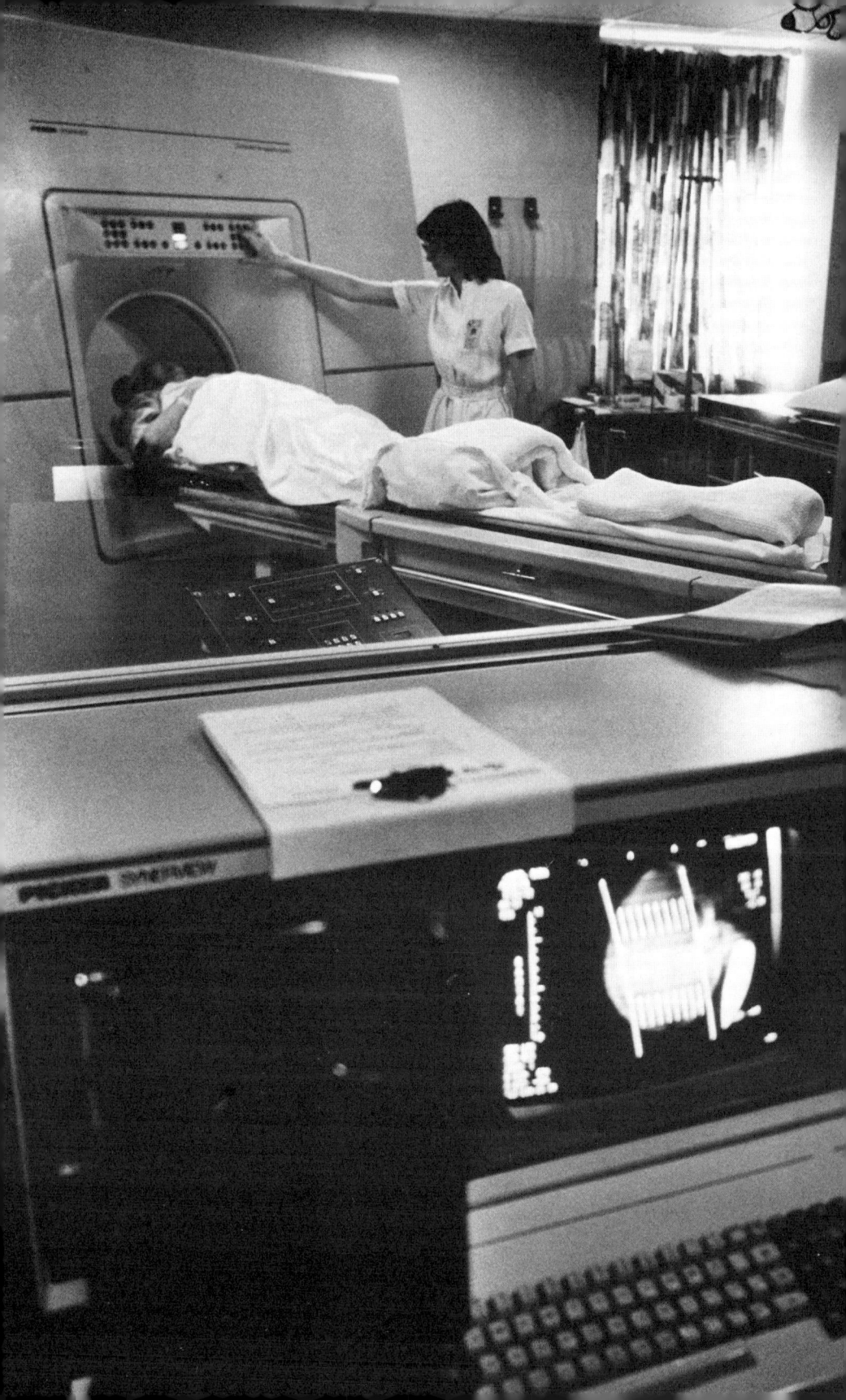

many hundred measurements of the X-ray transmission across the cross-sectional slice chosen in the patient. A typical scan takes from two to eight seconds, with more than seven-hundred-thousand measurements made per second. The mathematical process for reconstructing the image can be accomplished with times as fast as twelve to fourteen seconds.

How does the computer create an image from these thousands of measurements? Imagine a photograph of a slice of tissue, and superimpose a grid on top of it. Each volume element outlined by the grid is called a pixel, and the entire array is called a matrix. A series of X-ray beams are passed through the matrix from various positions around the tissue, and the fraction of the beam that is absorbed, called the CT number, is measured for each beam in every direction. The computer unscrambles this information and determines what the individual CT number of every pixel must have been to account for the observed absorption of each beam. The computer displays this array of pixels on a video screen, using varying shades of gray to represent the computed CT numbers. The resulting image can also be stored on magnetic tape or photographed for permanent record.

Images made with a CT scan are of extraordinary quality. Details of brain and spinal cord tissue, for example, can be made sharper and more detailed than ever before. The scan can detect certain tumors of the pituitary gland and other lesions that were almost impossible to visualize before.

The CT scanner gathers data through cross-sectional X rays which the computer then converts into a three-dimensional image.

DIGITAL SUBTRACTION ANGIOGRAPHY

The X-ray imaging of the body's circulatory system has been a very successful technique in detecting early symptoms of problems that might lead to heart attacks or strokes. One of the limitations of applying conventional X-rays to blood vessels, however, is that material other than bone shows up poorly on the film. In order to obtain a useful picture of the soft tissue of an artery, it is often necessary to introduce an absorbent material. The absorbent material, also called a contrast medium or dye, must concentrate in the vessel being examined and yet not be harmful. It must also strongly absorb X-rays so that the image of the organ being examined will stand out in sharp contrast from surrounding material. In the examination of arteries, for example, iodine is the most commonly used absorbing material.

Angiography is the technical name given to the procedure for producing an X-ray image of blood vessels—veins and arteries—that have been injected with a liquid contrast medium, such as iodine. It is used to help diagnose diseases of the circulatory system as well as the heart, kidneys, and other organs. Even with the addition of large amounts of contrast material, however, it is often difficult to see the blood vessels against the surrounding background material of bones and tissue.

Typically, a conventional angiogram is performed by inserting a small tube, or catheter, into a patient's artery and injecting an iodine dye. X-rays are taken and displayed on a fluoroscope, a device that has a video display similar to a television set. The process is complicated and uncomfortable for the patient. Puncturing an artery always involves some risk, and the procedure usually requires an overnight stay in the hospital. Also, the concentration of iodine required to obtain useful clinical information is high and can produce harmful side effects.

Most of these problems have been largely eliminated with the development of computerized digital subtraction angiography. The term *subtraction* refers to "subtracting the background," and the term *digital* refers to the digitizing of the image produced on the fluoroscope. A computer digitizes an image by subdividing it into small squares called pixels, and assigning a number to each pixel, a number that corresponds to that pixel's brightness. The images are read off the fluoroscope by a TV camera, digitized, and placed in the memory of a computer.

Digital subtraction angiography is extremely sensitive and uses concentrations of iodine that are some twenty times lower than in previous techniques. The greater sensitivity also permits the contrast medium to be injected into a patient's vein, typically in an arm or leg, rather than into an artery.

To start the procedure, X-rays are taken of the blood vessels before any contrasting medium is injected. These images are digitized and fed into a computer and will act as a reference, or "baseline." Iodine is then injected into the vein, and a second digitized image is obtained and stored in the computer. The computer then "subtracts" the image taken before the injection of the dye from the one taken after and creates a new image that displays only the veins or arteries filled with iodine. Unwanted structures that have not taken up the contrast medium, such as bone or overlapping organs, are screened out. The examining physician is presented with a highly detailed image of the blood vessel within seconds. The flow of injected iodine can also be followed as it passes through the arterial system. This is done by taking a series of X-rays at a rate as high as thirty pictures per second and subtracting the baseline from each.

For the patient, digital angiography means a faster, less invasive, and more comfortable diagnostic examination. Since less risk is associated with digital angiography, it can be performed as an outpatient procedure, avoiding the costs of a hospital stay. And the results can be stored in the computer for later study.

ULTRASONOGRAPHY

One of the safest and least invasive methods of imaging the body makes use of high-frequency ultrasound waves similar to those associated with sonar. In this technique, short ultrasonic pulses and their echoes are used to probe the soft tissues of the body and produce images that will detect abnormalities. This procedure is particularly valuable for the examination of pregnant women and children since there is no involvement with any ionizing radiation such as X-rays. A variety of body functions, such as the performance of the heart and the flow of blood, can be studied. Various diseases and abnormalities, such as cancer, tumors, and cysts can be identified.

The ultrasound pulses are created by a special crytalline material called a piezoelectric crystal. This crystal has the remarkable ability to vibrate mechanically when a varying electrical signal is applied to it. In turn, it produces a varying electrical signal when it is mechanically vibrated so that it can be used both as a transmitter and receiver. The piezoelectric crystal may be familiar to you as the device connected to a phonograph needle that changes the needle's motion, generated by the record's grooves, into sound.

The doctor usually places the ultrasonic probe, which looks like a large pen, against the patient's skin. To maximize the transmission of the sound into the body it is generally "coupled" to the skin through a layer of special oil or gel; this cuts down on energy losses. The probe, which also acts as the detector, contains the piezoelectric transmitter and a lens to focus the emerging beam. The beam consists of a series of ultrasonic pulses that are emitted about a thousandth of a second apart.

The ultrasonic pulses generated by the piezoelectric

transmitter are far above the range of human hearing, with frequencies of four to seven million vibrations per second. The frequency range of ordinary audible sound is much lower, from about forty to twenty thousand vibrations per second.

As the ultra-high frequency sound travels through the body, some of the energy carried by the pulse is reflected and scattered. This happens whenever the sound travels across an interface or boundary between different types of tissue. At the boundary between kidney tissue and fat tissue, for example, approximately one half of one percent of the sound pulse is reflected. The partial reflection is caused by changes in tissue density. In this way organs can be outlined by the echoes bounced off their boundaries. As the ultrasonic pulse makes its way through the body, it may reach the front wall of some organ and produce an echo. Most of the original pulse continues through the organ, though, and eventually reaches the back wall, where a second echo is produced. The remainder of the pulse can continue on to be reflected by other structures. Detecting these echoes supplies information about the position of the reflecting interfaces in the body.

Ultrasonography depends on precise measurements of the time intervals between the transmitted sound pulses and the echoes. This information is fed into a computer, which can produce several types of display. In one variation, the echo strength is presented on a screen plotted as a function of time. Since the time it takes the pulse to arrive at a certain point within the body and to return is directly related to the distance traveled by the pulse, the time scale is, in effect, a measurement of location within the body. This permits the physician to precisely locate certain structures within the body. The absence of an echo at a certain point on the time scale can also be meaningful. The lack of an echo from a region where one is expected might indicate the presence of a cyst whose liquid content, unlike solid tissue, returns practically no echoes.

Cross-sections of the body can also be generated by a series of scans at different angles. This is often done to monitor the progress of a fetus before birth. In this type of scan, each ultrasonic echo is represented by a spot of light. The brightness of the spot represents the strength of the echo, and its position represents the position of the reflecting boundary. The ultrasonic probe is placed on the abdomen of a pregnant woman, for example, and moved in a straight line from one side of the abdomen to the other. As its position is changed, the probe sends out pulses and receives echoes from many different locations along its path. The position and brightness of all the echoes are stored in the memory of a computer. At the end of the series of measurements, the computer digitizes and adds up the information from each scan and displays it as a cross-section of the fetus made in a particular plane through the mother's body. The brain and internal organs of the fetus are often clearly revealed.

A recent development in the treatment of heart disease uses ultrasound to diagnose diseases of the heart valves and arteries. After being reflected from various locations on the heart, the echoes are processed by a computer to display pictures of the beating heart on a video display. Physicians can actually observe the valves and chambers of the heart as it pumps blood through the body.

COMPUTERIZED RADIATION THERAPY

The use of radiation for the treatment of various types of tumors is well known. The success of the therapy depends on careful planning by the physician. With radiation as a medical tool used so frequently today, it is extremely important to avoid the damage to healthy tissue that radiation can cause. In many cases, such damage could in itself be fatal. The amount of radiation to be administered, and where it is to be localized and for how long, are all decisions that will affect the success of the treatment.

Radiation therapists need accurate information about the anatomy of the patient. They need to know exactly where the tumor is and how large it is. In the past, much of this information came from ordinary X-rays. During the last decade, though, ultrasonography and computed tomography have contributed significantly to supplying more exact data for the treatment.

Computers have recently been used to plan exact radiation doses, doing complex X-ray and electron beam calculations that would be almost impossible to manage by hand. An X-ray is first taken of the area to be treated. The information is then conveyed to a computer by tracing the outline of the treatment area with a penlike instrument connected to the computer. The computer then creates a diagram of the patient and plans an optimum method of treatment showing exactly how much radiation will be deposited in neighboring tissue.

COMPUTERIZED DIAGNOSIS OF HEART DISEASE

Computers are being used at the North Shore University Hospital on Long Island to diagnose heart disease—without the aid of conventional electrocardiograms or stress tests. Making use of a technique developed by Dr. John Morrison, director of North Shore's Coronary Care Unit, computers at the hospital can detect heart problems early enough to treat them more effectively.

Physicians initiate the test by injecting a radioactive isotope called thallium-201 into the patient. Although the thallium is only mildly radioactive and presents no hazard in itself, it does give off gamma rays as it disintegrates within the body. These gamma rays strongly resemble X-rays in their properties and can be detected outside the body by a gamma scintillation camera.

As the radioactive substance passes through the heart, the thallium-201 is taken up only by healthy heart cells and tissue. It is rejected by dying or dead cells. The gamma scintillation camera is then positioned over the patient's chest, where it detects the radiation from the thallium that has adhered to the heart. This information is given to a computer that creates an image of the heart on a video screen. Any damage to the heart can be clearly seen. The images are usually in color, with healthy tissue displayed in white or yellow and dying or dead tissue in orange or red. The physician can see the extent of heart damage at a glance and immediately initiate proper treatment.

NUCLEAR MAGNETIC RESONANCE

Nuclear magnetic resonance (NMR) is one of the newest imaging techniques available to physicians. It can obtain cross-sectional pictures of the body without exposing the patient to ionizing radiation and can discriminate between healthy and diseased tissue with greater sensitivity and accuracy than any other available technique. Many questions remain unanswered about NMR's clinical applicability, but results so far seem to indicate that it will prove to be a powerful diagnostic tool.

In this technique, the patient is inserted into a body-size chamber similar to the gantry used in CT. The chamber houses electric coils that can produce magnetic fields as high as fifteen thousand gauss, some thirty thousand times stronger than the earth's magnetic field. This magnetic field causes the nuclei of certain atoms in the body to align themselves in the magnetic field.

Some nuclei, namely those with an odd number of protons and neutrons, can be thought of as behaving like tiny, spinning particles. Hydrogen, with only one proton in its nucleus, is an important example. The human body is seventy-five percent water, each molecule of which contains two atoms of hydrogen. Because nuclei are electrically charged, their spin produces a magnetic field similar to a little bar magnet or compass, with a north and south pole. When placed in a magnetic field, these nuclei will orient themselves in the field in a fashion similar to a compass.

The gantry surrounding the patient contains equipment for broadcasting radio frequency signals. When such a signal is sent out at just the right frequency, it can cause the nuclei to absorb enough energy to reverse their spins. When the radio frequency field is turned off, the nuclei revert back to their original spin direction, re-emitting the energy they originally absorbed. This energy, called the NMR signal, is detected by a receiver contained in the gantry. The NMR signal depends on the local chemical environment of the nucleus being probed and on the number of nuclei present.

Further information about the spatial position of the NMR signal is obtained by adding a gradient to the applied magnetic field. A gradient means simply that the field varies in strength inside the gantry rather than being the same throughout the entire chamber. The NMR signal will have characteristics that depend on where in the gradient the nucleus happens to be. Data from the receiver is fed into a computer, which computes individual pixel values and displays an image on a TV monitor. The image can either be in gray scale or color and can be photographed for permanent storage and interpretation.

It is expected that NMR imaging will be able to help physicians distinguish between benign and malignant tumors, detect conditions that may lead to heart attacks and strokes, and assess conditions involving muscles. NMR has already defined certain changes in the brain associated with multiple sclerosis better than CT scans. One of the outstanding capabilities of NMR is its potential to probe body chemistry in a living person.

PET—POSITRON EMISSION TOMOGRAPHY

Imagine being able to watch the brain think and feel. A new technique that uses a radioactive isotope that emits a positive electron, or positron, allows doctors to actually observe the brain perform these functions. This new method is called PET, for positron emission tomography, or occasionally PETT, for positron emission transaxial tomography. It is rapidly becoming one of the most important tools for diagnosis available to physicians.

From a distance, a PET scanner looks very much like a CT imager. There is a large metal gantry that surrounds the patient, containing hundreds of radiation detectors arranged on rings. Nearby are magnetic disks, a line printer, and a video display system. Unlike a CT scan, however, this procedure will "see" radiation that originates inside the patient. The radiation consists of gamma rays that are formed when the positron given off by a previously injected radioisotope collides with an ordinary electron. The positron and electron "annihilate" each other during this collision, and their mass is transformed into two gamma rays that are emitted "back-to-back," that is, in diametrically opposite directions. The detectors are arranged so that they will record an event only when two detectors opposite each other on the ring simultaneously receive a gamma ray. An event of this kind defines a line through the patient along which the "annihilation" took place. Thousands of these events are recorded, and the data is given to a computer, which reconstructs the positions and distribution of the positrons in the body.

Radioactive atoms are introduced into the patient's body by making them part of a chemical or biological compound that is used or metabolized by the body. Sugar is one of the most common substances "labeled" in this way. The labeled substance is introduced into the body, and the patient is scanned with radiation detectors to see where the labeled substance goes. It accumulates in areas that are taking up and using the compound. Brain tissues actively absorb sugar when they are thinking and feeling so that the radioactively tagged sugar becomes a tracer that clearly "lights up" the precise area of the brain that is doing the work.

The positron-emitting isotopes most useful for labeling in PET studies are carbon 11, nitrogen 13, and fluorine 18. Unfortunately, these are all very short-lived radioisotopes. The carbon has a half-life of twenty minutes, the nitrogen a half-life of ten minutes, and the fluorine a half-life of two hours. The radioactive fluorine, for example, is usually incorporated into a glucose molecule to measure the sugar uptake in the brain. The labeled sugar is called FDG, an acronym of its chemical formula 18F-2-fluoro-2-deoxyglucose. After a period of only four or five hours, the FDG has lost too much of its radioactivity to be of any value. This tight time restraint means that the large and very expensive cyclotrons and linear accelerators that are used to produce the isotopes must be very close to the hospital engaged in PET studies. Scientists must also devise extremely rapid chemical procedures for introducing the radioactive labels into useful biological compounds.

One of the first measurements made with a PET scanner was that of the blood volume in the brain of a normal man. The patient inhaled air that had small amounts of carbon monoxide labeled with carbon 11. The carbon monoxide attached itself to the hemoglobin in the blood and was quickly carried throughout the body. PET images made of sections of the brain clearly showed the regions of high blood volume.

The use of PET scans is being explored as a research tool in the study of metabolism in various parts of the body, as well as a means to map areas of the heart that have been damaged by a heart attack. It is in the study of the brain, however, that PET has made its greatest contributions. Glucose metabolism studies comparing the

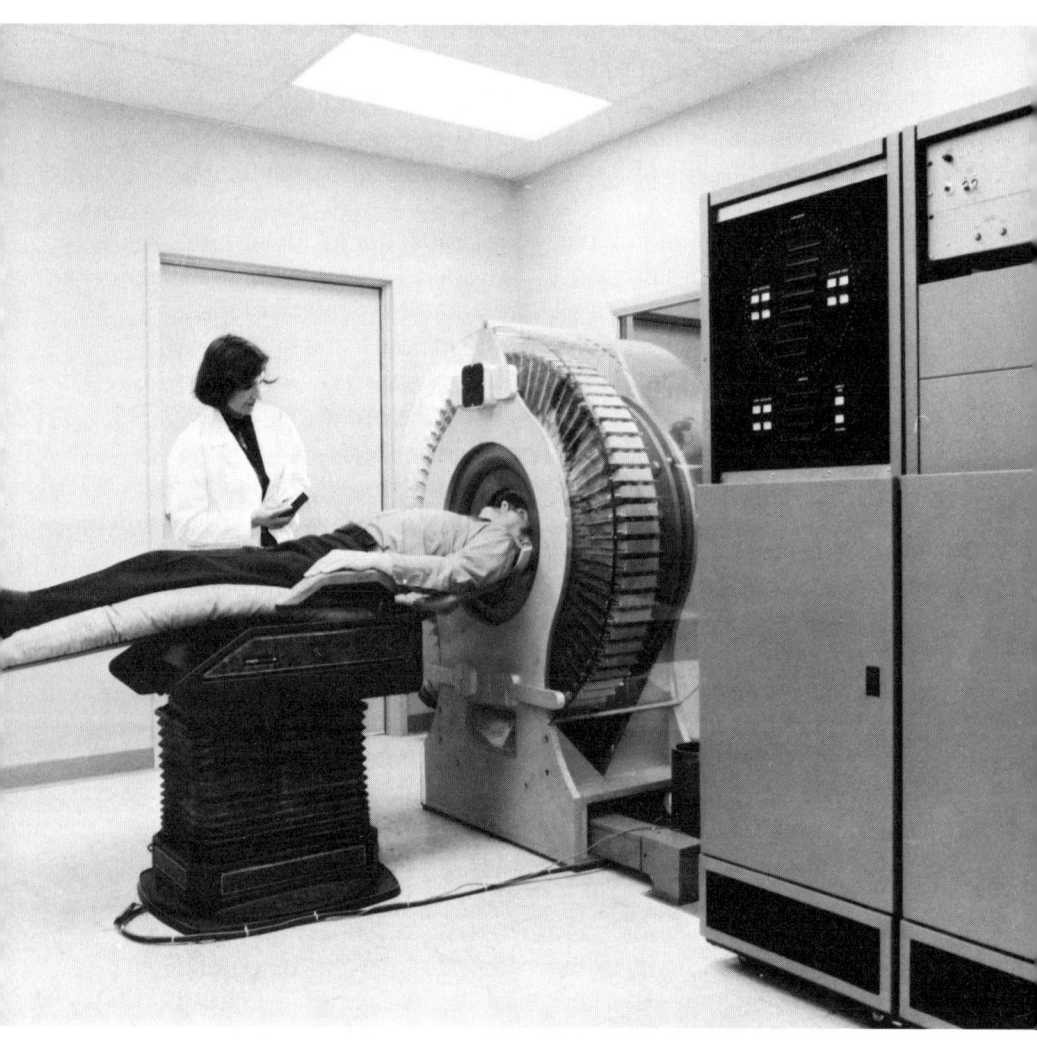

The PET scanner (above) makes it possible to actually observe the workings of the human brain. At right are computer images of brain scans from a normal person, a depressed person, and a schizophrenic that were taken at Brookhaven National Laboratory as part of a study on the correlation between glucose metabolism and brain dysfunction.

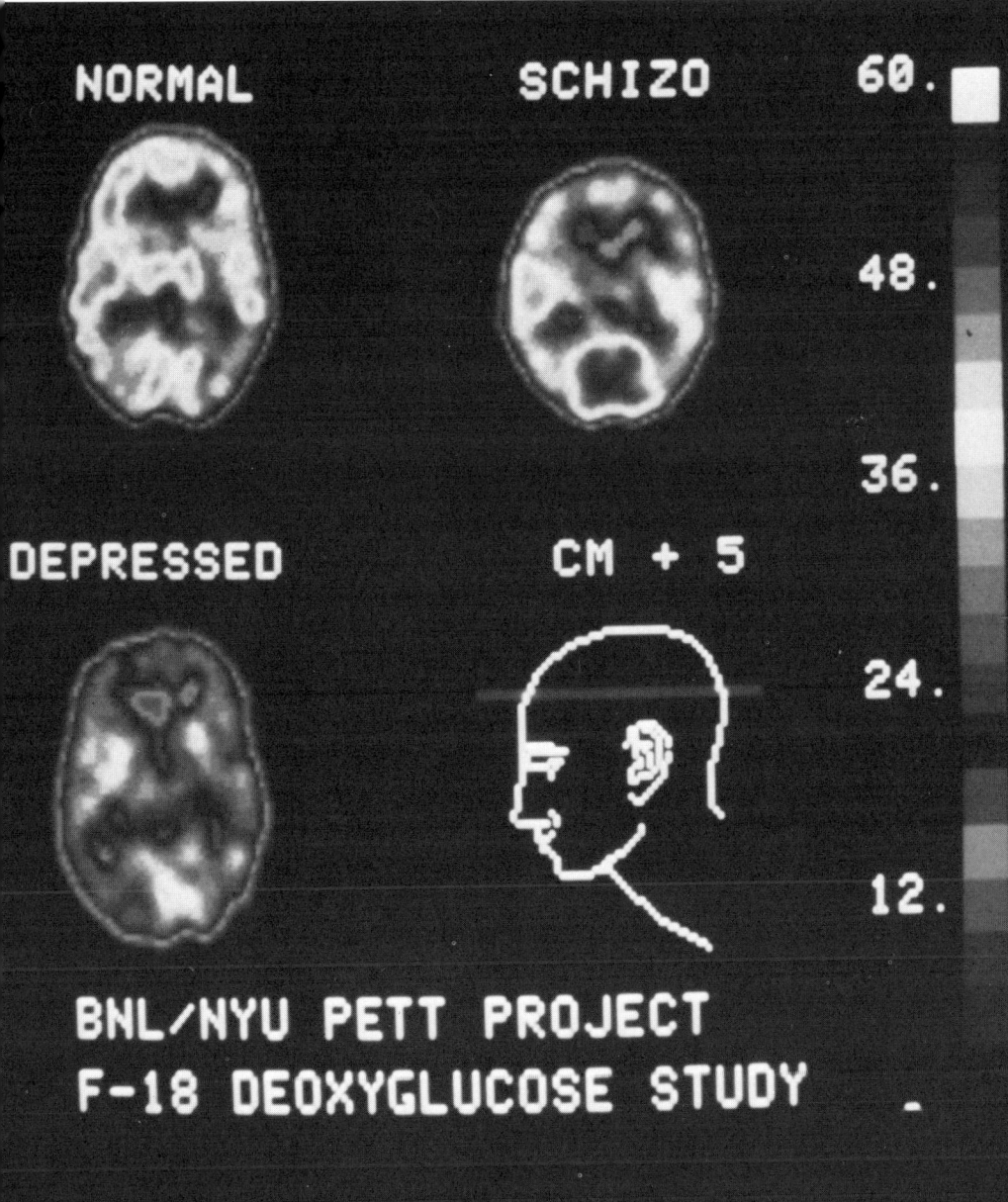

brains of normal subjects with those suffering from Alzheimer's disease, a disorder associated with memory loss, are being carried out at New York University Medical Center.

At Brookhaven National Laboratory, Dr. Alfred P. Wolf and his colleagues are using glucose uptake to study the brain during different activities and states of mind. In one experiment Dr. Wolf, using himself as a subject, listened to music while undergoing a PET scan. In his own words, the pictures made by the computer of the left hemisphere of his brain lighted up "like a neon light." The PET promises to lead to many new discoveries about the brain. Recently, Dr. Wolf's group joined with researchers at the New York University Medical Center to study glucose metabolism in different regions of the brain as it relates to aging, senile dementia, and schizophrenia.

CHAPTER 5

MORE TOOLS FOR DIAGNOSIS

Symptoms of illness are often puzzling. Why is Mr. Schwartz running a fever? What is the reason for little Jenny Lun's vomiting spells? The more information doctors can obtain on a patient's condition, the better their chances of making a correct diagnosis and quickly starting the right treatment.

Accuracy is one reason for using computer-aided diagnostic tools. Speed and efficiency is another. Yet another reason is that computerized diagnosis can sometimes save a patient the discomfort of more invasive tests.

RADIOLOGY

Not all diagnostic examinations require computerized instruments, of course. Still, laboratories using traditional instruments work with greater speed and efficiency when they are organized using computerized record keeping.

A diagnostic radiology department, for example, becomes a model of automated efficiency with the help of a central computer. An X-ray technologist positions the patient and takes the required number of pictures. A technician then develops the negatives, brings them to the radiologist's office, and slides them into lighted wall panels that illuminate all details clearly from the back. The radiologist examines the X-rays while dictating the findings through a telephone onto a tape. In another part of the hospital, a typist sitting before a computer terminal listens to the tape through earphones and enters the doctor's report into the computer. The typist is able to do this very quickly, by combining code words that call up standard prewritten texts with the doctor's special observations on the case.

BLOOD CHEMISTRY

More hospital tests are done on blood than are done on any other biological substance. Hospital laboratories analyze hundreds of blood samples a day. Some tests are done as part of routine checkups or in preparation for surgery. Others are done to investigate disorders of the liver or kidneys, as well as infections and many other kinds of illness. At times, blood tests must be rushed through in minutes, for patients in the emergency room or on the operating table.

Blood is a complicated substance. It contains formed elements, as well as water and many different chemicals in solution. The formed elements consist of red blood cells, white blood cells, and platelets. The red blood cells carry oxygen from the lungs to all the organs and take back carbon dioxide for the lungs to exhale. The white cells help the body fight infection. The platelets are involved in blood clotting. As for the dissolved chemicals, their quantity and proportions may indicate numerous imbalances and disorders.

BLOOD GAS

A young man is rushed to the emergency room, unconscious. Is he suffering from a drug overdose? A diabetic condition? A blow on the head? The answer depends in part on the proportion of oxygen to carbon dioxide in the patient's blood, and on its acidity. A severe imbalance in blood gases can mean that not enough oxygen is reaching the patient's organs. This can rapidly become fatal. Treatment must begin quickly, and the right treatment depends on the right diagnosis.

To analyze blood gases, a sample of blood is taken from the patient's artery and dispatched to the laboratory through a pneumatic tube. Since quick results are essential, hospitals with a central computer have a great advantage. The emergency room nurse need only type the rush order on the terminal. The printer automatically types out a form to accompany the vial of blood, giving the patient's identification number, the code number of the emergency room, the type of test needed, and the time. A priority order comes clattering out of the laboratory printer. The moment the blood has arrived, the laboratory technologist places the sample in the blood gas analyzer. Within seconds, this instrument transmits its results to the computer. At the other end of the hospital, doctors in the emergency room can read the test results simply by glancing at the CRT screen.

SMAC

A very important instrument in the chemistry laboratory is the Sequential Multiple Analyzer Computer, or SMAC. Using only half a milliliter of blood serum, SMAC can detect the presence and quantity of components such as blood sugar, cholesterol, protein, and albumen, as well as of electrolytes such as sodium, potassium, and chloride. Doctors can order tests for as few as one or two of these substances or for as many as twenty. They can also ask

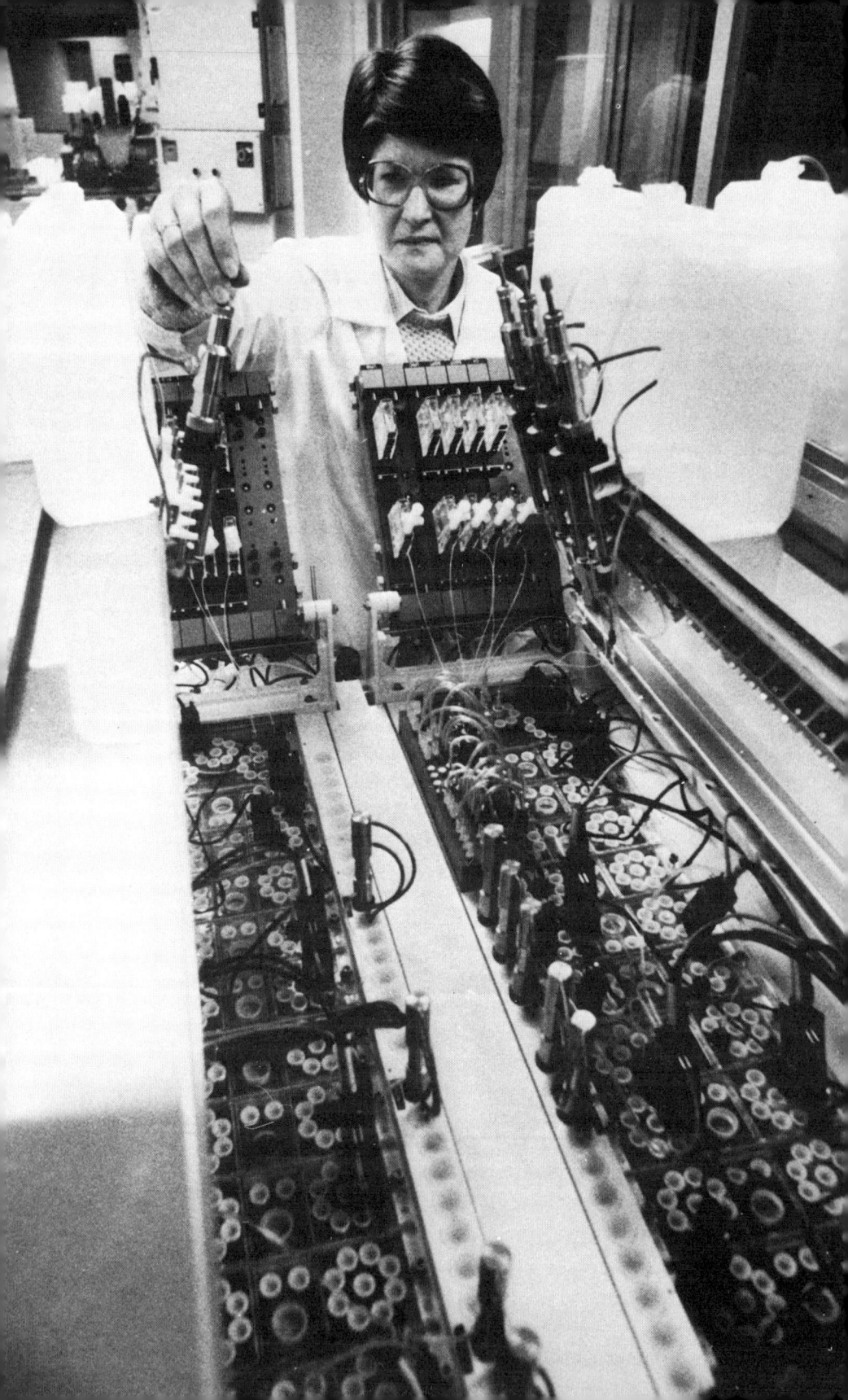

for the particular set of tests that reveal a patient's "liver profile" or kidney functioning. SMAC is so efficient that it can handle a hundred and fifty samples an hour in a continuous flow.

Blood plasma is brought to SMAC in a carrier of test tubes, each with a patient identification number on a little card. An electronic lamp reads the number while a probe draws a sample of about five milliliters up a riser column by means of a pump. The plasma goes through tubes and is divided up and delivered to a number of analytical cartridges. In each cartridge, the sample is mixed with a reagent, which causes it to become colored. Then it passes through to a colorimeter.

The colorimeter can determine the concentration of a particular substance by measuring how much light it absorbs in a specified color range. These findings are converted into electrical signals and transmitted to the computer, where they are printed out in readable form and stored in the memory.

SMAC is programmed to time itself, monitor itself, calibrate itself, and even to wash its own tubes and channels. If it encounters any highly unusual reading, it sounds an alarm. It also rings for help from its supervisor when dust or a clot enter its tubing or when it starts to run out of reagent.

This machine, called PRISMA (Programmable Individually Selective Modular Analyzer), is capable of testing 300 blood specimens per hour, performing 25 analyses on each one.

HEMATRAK

Artificial intelligence (AI) is a branch of computer science that develops machines capable of making judgments and decisions. The most "intelligent" of the automatic analyzers in the chemistry laboratory is Hematrak. Its specialty is the "differential" count of white blood cells. This term refers to the proportion of normal to abnormal white cells in a patient's blood. Usually, one hundred or two hundred cells are counted. The results are then given as percentages of the different types of white blood cells present.

Before Hematrak was brought into the lab, a technologist used to count white cells by examining a blood smear on a slide under a microscope. This was a time-consuming process. Hematrak works much like its human counterpart, only faster. It also has the ability to compare new cell shapes to shapes already present in its memory— a technique known as pattern recognition. By means of microscope optics, Hematrak scans the blood smear through a digitizing color video scanner. This means that it senses shapes and patterns by their light densities, to which it then assigns numerical values.

Each time Hematrak finds a white cell, it transmits the digitized image to its image memory. Here, it keeps digital records of many different kinds of normal white blood cells. If the machine can "recognize" the new cell by matching it to one of these patterns, it classifies and adds it to the count.

Whenever the machine cannot exactly match a cell to its stored patterns, it makes a tentative classification, stops scanning, and rings a bell. The technician then looks through a microscope viewer to identify the cell that has puzzled Hematrak. If the machine's classification is incorrect, the technician enters the correct one on the keyboard. After computing its final results, Hematrak displays its findings on the CRT screen and prints them on a form. It can also send them to a central computer.

ACCURACY CONTROLS

One more marvelous feature of the computerized instruments in the blood chemistry lab is that they are programmed to keep themselves in top condition. Periodically, each instrument goes through a complete check of its own tubes and channels—in fact, its entire system. Then it goes through a chemistry check. It knows what readings it should get from a standard sample and calibrates itself accordingly. Computers are also used to compare the accuracy of results obtained by hospitals and clinical laboratories all over the United States.

EVOKED POTENTIALS

All sights, sounds, and feelings are transmitted to the brain by pathways of nerve cells, or neurons. When a neuron in a fingertip, for instance, comes in contact with an ice cube, it emits a signal that stimulates the neuron adjacent to it. This neuron, in turn, stimulates its neighbor to pass the signal further, and so on up the line. In this way, the impulse travels along the nerve trunk until it reaches the brain. All stimuli to the body are transmitted the same way. What differs is the part of the brain to which each organ sends its impulses for interpretation.

In normal subjects, nerve impulses travel from stimulus to brain in milliseconds. But if the pathway is blocked, impulses travel slowly or not at all. This may be due to brain, spinal cord, or muscular diseases. By monitoring the time it takes for impulses to reach the brain from different parts of the body, neurologists can diagnose conditions such as multiple sclerosis and many other disorders.

The traditional test for brain activity is the EEG (electroencephalogram), which records brainwaves—the patterns of oscillating electrical activity in the brain. So much goes on in the brain at any given moment, though, that responses from stimuli to one area cannot be distinguished from the overall action. It takes the computer's powers of digital analysis to subtract background "noise" and to sort out, amplify and keep track of a particular sequence of stimuli and responses. The computer then compares the results with a set of responses considered normal either in the general population or in the particular patient's past history.

Testing for evoked potentials is usually done as a series of three procedures. All are non-invasive and painless. In the first, the patient, wearing three electrodes attached to the scalp, is seated before a visual stimulus. It may be a screen showing black and white squares or a sequence of light flashes. One eye at a time is tested, while the other eye is covered by a patch. The computer calculates and records the time it takes the stimulus to reach the occipital lobe of the brain. While recording numerical data, the computer also projects waves of neuron activity on the CRT screen. The screen can show a few hundred waveforms at a time.

An hour-long brain stem test follows. This is an auditory test. Again, electrodes are placed on the patient's scalp, but on a different portion of it. This time, also, the patient is lying down in a darkened room. The stimulus is a series of loud clicking sounds.

The last test measures somatosensory response. The somatosensory cortex is the region of the brain that receives impulses from all the general sense receptors of the skin, impulses such as pressure, touch, and pain. Now, the stimulus is a mild electric current applied to different parts of the body. In examining a partly paralyzed accident victim, for example, the computer might be used to measure the time it takes impulses to travel from the affected limb to the spinal cord. In some cases, early waves may be recorded but then drop out at the level of midbrain without reaching their destination.

Evoked potentials can be used to detect hearing defects in babies and small children because the tests do not require active participation from the patient. Evoked potentials can even be tested on patients in coma, to assess what stimuli are successful in reaching the brain.

NON-INVASIVE TESTS

One of the best things about computer-aided diagnosis is that it can often be carried out painlessly and safely, without any surgical invasion of the body. We have already shown several examples, including various types of scanning and evoked potentials.

Recently, a way to save chronically ill patients the pain of a certain test for iron deficiency was reported in a medical journal. Ordinarily, the test for iron requires surgical extraction of a sample of the patient's bone marrow. Now, researchers have developed a way to predict the presence of iron in the bone marrow by a sequence of five blood tests. Using complex statistical methods based on mathematical probability theory, the computer quickly accomplishes what laboratory staff members would have had to spend many hours figuring out. It calculates the likelihood that the subject is iron deficient. Only if the probability is very high—above ninety-five percent—is the actual sampling of bone marrow recommended, to obtain certainty. The computer has eliminated the need for the painful procedure in ninety-six percent of all cases.

In the future, doctors expect to use mathematical probability calculated by computer more often to help them make diagnoses and crucial decisions concerning tests, treatment, and surgery.

CHAPTER 6

INTENSIVE CARE

Patients who are critically ill need constant close observation. Their vital functions are delicately balanced and can deteriorate in a very short time. The smallest change can quickly lead to disaster.

James Masaro, a fifty-two-year-old heavy smoker, is recovering from complications of his diabetic condition. His vital signs have been stable for the past twenty-four hours. Now, however, a nurse making a routine check notices that his skin is very pale and moist. He complains of chest pains, and his answers to questions are confused. His breathing is rapid and labored. His blood pressure has taken a sudden drop.

The doctor in charge, having rushed to the bedside, diagnoses cardiogenic shock. He orders oxygen and intravenous medication for the patient and gives instructions to rush him to the hospital's intensive care unit (ICU) without delay.

Cardiogenic shock—shock originating from the

heart—is sometimes referred to as pump failure. Usually, it is not the entire heart that fails but the left ventricle—the part that pumps oxygenated blood into the aorta and from there through arteries to the rest of the body. When the pumping of the heat is weak, not enough oxygenated blood reaches the body's tissues. Without oxygen, tissues quickly deteriorate. The body reacts to a drop in heart output by drawing blood away from the extremities and the brain toward the inner organs. Unless blood flow is restored immediately, the condition quickly leads to death.

A modern ICU is arranged so that six or eight cubicles with beds facing outward are placed opposite a nursing station in full view of the desk. Above each bed, a microprocessor unit with a CRT screen is attached to the wall or to a stand. This small computer will be Mr. Masaro's guardian during the next few days and nights. The patient's vital functions, such as his heart rate, blood pressure, and temperature, will be measured by various probes that lead from his body to the computer. Sensors in the probes convert forms of energy, such as pressure, heat, or light, into electrical impulses. When these impulses are transmitted to the computer, it analyzes the information and presents it in easy-to-read form on the screen. It also stores the information for future reference.

The monitor unit accommodates several removable modules, each designed to measure a different bodily function. A typical intensive care bedside monitor may be equipped with modules to measure heartbeat, body temperature, venous and arterial blood pressure, blood loss, and urine output.

THE COMPUTERIZED ELECTROCARDIOGRAM

One of the vital signs that the computer above Mr. Masaro's bed will monitor continuously is his electrocardiogram, or ECG (pronounced Eee-Kay-Gee). The ECG is a recording of waveforms produced by the electrical signals given off by the beating heart. The ECG recording instrument has twelve leads ending in small suction cups. The nurse places these on the patient's chest, arms, and legs. Electrodes pick up the heart signals. The waves of a normal ECG are regular and basically unchanging. Electronic sensors detect even tiny changes in the rhythms of the heart cycle.

In the past, arrythmias—premature or missing beats—were the number one cause of death for heart patients. But the only way to observe them was by the human eye. Nurses had to take turns, around the clock, observing the wave patterns of the patient's ECG as it was recorded on a long roll of graph paper. An experienced nurse can detect about eighty-five percent of irregularities. A computer, though, picks up about ninety percent.

Mr. Masaro's ECG, which is continuously displayed on the CRT screen above his bed, also appears on a screen at the nursing desk outside the room. This master screen can show the ECG patterns of six patients at the same time. The computer is programmed for pattern recognition. It has a digitized memory of each patient's regular heartbeat. Against this pattern, it constantly matches the new wave patterns as they appear. If it detects a skipped beat, rhythmic changes, or a weakening of the signal, it sends an alarm to the nurses' desk. Though it "freezes" the irregular tracing on the upper part of the screen for a nurse to examine, it continues recording on the lower half of the screen. It saves the irregular episodes and stores them in a separate part of its memory.

A doctor making the morning rounds who wants to see what the patient's heart activity was during the night need only press a few keys to obtain a display or printed readout of all the irregular episodes that occurred during the previous eight hours. Have irregular episodes increased or decreased in frequency and number? The computer pro-

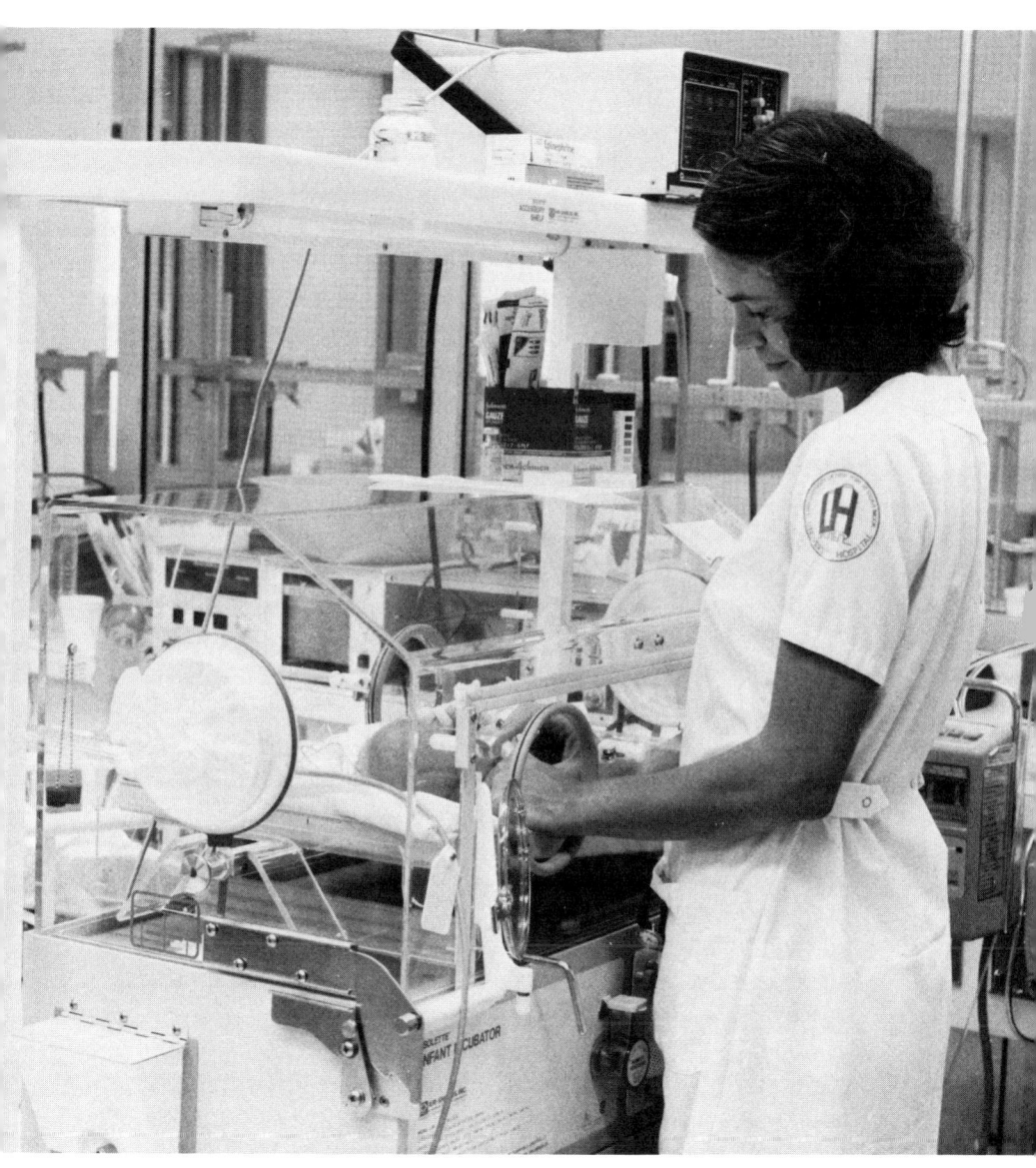

Computer-assisted monitoring devices, among them the ECG machine on the shelf, are used in this intensive care unit for the newborn.

vides figures analyzing the trend. It can also enlarge any part of the pattern for closer study or make it smaller for an overall view. Next to the nursing desk, a printer, connected to the computer, can produce a readout on paper of the patterns, to be placed in the patient's permanent file.

MEASURING CARDIAC OUTPUT

The electrocardiogram is an external, non-invasive measurement of the heartbeat. For greater precision, though, doctors can observe the heart directly by inserting thin, flexible tubes called catheters into the major veins and arteries. Each catheter is inserted through a small incision, either at the patient's wrists, near the groin, or at the neck. Through the catheters, tiny precision instruments sense the pressure in each part of the pumping heart and send this information to the computer in electronic form. Here, again, the electrical impulses are digitized, analyzed, displayed in wave form, and stored for later recall. The computer's ability to recognize abnormal patterns allows it to respond to an emergency and to flash an alarm signal to the nursing station.

Because the body's organs and extremities need a constant blood supply, the amount of blood the heart pumps out with each beat is a crucial health factor. The cardiac index—a formula for heart output per square meter of body surface—helps determine how well a heart patient is responding to therapy.

Two methods for direct measurement of heart output are made possible by the computer. The first method produces a time-based dye concentration curve. A nurse injects a measured quantity of harmless dye through the catheter into the right atrium of the patient's heart. This upper heart chamber receives the blood from the veins and pushes it out again through the arteries, by way of the lungs, to all parts of the body. As the heart pumps the dye-stained blood, samples are steadily withdrawn from the patient's arteries and passed through a light-sensitive instrument called a densitometer. The densitometer, in turn, is connected to the computer. The computer calculates the heart's output according to the dye concentration and the time it takes for the dye to disperse.

A second method for measuring cardiac output uses a low temperature liquid instead of a dye. In this test, too, the doctor advances a catheter into the right atrium. This catheter, though, ends in a tiny balloon. When the balloon is inflated with about a milliliter of air, the current of the blood carries it forward into the pulmonary artery. Once it lodges there, the balloon is deflated. At the outer end, the catheter terminates in several ports. One port is used to inflate the balloon, another to insert liquids, and still another to measure the temperature of the liquids as they mix with the patient's blood.

The nurse takes the patient's temperature rectally and dials it into the computer. Some bedside monitors include a rectal probe thermometer with direct computer input. Near the bed, a sterile saline solution is kept under refrigeration at a temperature between zero and five degrees centigrade. Just before injecting the solution, the nurse dials the exact temperature and quantity of the solution into the computer. Very rapidly, now, the cold solution is injected through the special catheter into the right atrium. The resulting temperature changes in the pulmonary artery are read by a thermistor—a temperature-sensitive resistor—with input to the computer. The computer is programmed to calculate the rate of temperature change and convert it into the cardiac output figure.

Such invasive tests are not without danger. They may stop the heart altogether or else cause it to go into cramp-like motions called fibrillation, that prevent it from pumping any blood. If this occurs, the computer sounds an alarm and red lights flash at the nurses' station. The hospital's cardiac rescue team rushes to the scene. Part of the computer's equipment may be a so-called heart clock above the patient's bed. Its hand begins to move when the heart stops so that rescuers can tell how long the heart has been inactive. This information helps them assess how much damage may have been done to the patient's brain before they succeeded in restoring the heartbeat.

MONITORING OTHER VITAL SIGNS

In the cubicle next to Mr. Masaro's lies a young construction worker who was seriously injured two days earlier when a steel girder accidentally dropped from a hoist. He is recovering from a skull fracture and concussion. The computer above his bed monitors not only his pulse rate, blood pressure, and temperature but also measures his intracranial pressure. This is the pressure exerted by the brain, blood, and cerebrospinal fluid on the skull. Increased pressure can cause brain damage and death.

It is difficult to assess intracranial pressure by external observation. Instead, doctors bore a small hole in the patient's skull and insert a photocell sensor in the space between the skull and the surface of the brain. The pressure measurements are relayed from the sensor to the computer. The monitor above the bed displays intracranial pressure in waves that relate to changes in the patient's breathing and blood circulation.

Respiration is another vital function that computers are called on to monitor in intensive care. The computer is especially needed by patients who cannot get enough air breathing on their own. When this happens, a carefully regulated stream of air must be supplied to the lungs through a tube in the patient's nose or through a surgical opening in the patient's windpipe. The computer supervises the patient's inhalation as well as exhalation. The exhaled gases are channeled to pass by an infrared sensor connected to the microprocessor. The sensor detects carbon dioxide and water vapor in the patient's breath for the purpose of measuring respiratory rate and tidal volume—or how rapidly and deeply the patient breathes and how many cubic centimeters of air he or she delivers with each breath.

The computer regulates the air supply according to the patient's needs. It records changes in airway pressure, and unusually high or low readings trip an alarm. For absolute safety, the machine was built with many checks and balances, to prevent any malfunctioning and accidents, such as leaky or detached tubes.

When patients begin to recover, they must be weaned away from dependence on the respirator. To encourage the patient's lungs to expand and contract normally, the artificial air supply is adjusted to a necessary minimum. As the computer senses the growing strength of the patient's breathing, it provides less and less artificial help until the patient is able to breathe independently.

TELEMETRY

After Mr. Masaro has recovered from his heart attack he will be able to go home, provided he takes medication to regulate his heartbeat. Precise doses of drugs for heart arrythmias need frequent adjusting, so Mr. Masaro will probably return to the hospital for observation a few months later. This time, though, he will not be confined to a bed. He will walk around, chat with people, and eat normal meals while his ECG is being monitored by telemetry, a technique for monitoring the heart from a distance. Slung across his chest like a camera bag, Mr. Masaro will carry around the wireless telemetry unit. This instrument picks up the electrical signals of his heartbeat and relays their wave patterns to the desktop computer at the nursing station, for display and recording.

CHAPTER 7

RESEARCH THROUGH DATA BANKS AND COMPUTER MODELING

On July 14, 1966, twenty-four-year-old Richard Speck forced his way at knife and gun point into a Chicago nurse's residence. There, he strangled eight student nurses, one of whom he also raped. When the police caught up with him, they discovered that he had been arrested thirty-seven times for previous offenses. Speck wore the legend "Born to Raise Hell" tattooed on his left forearm. During the trial, his defense attorneys attempted to show that their client was not accountable for his crimes because of an inherited genetic defect. He was, in fact, born with two male sex chromosomes instead of one. The lawyers claimed that the extra male chromosome had made this huge, gangling man aggressive beyond his own control.

Normally, both men and women have two chromosomes each. Women have two X-chromosomes (XX), men have an X and a Y (XY) chromosome. A simple test on a few skin cells can give doctors a complete picture of any patient's chromosomes. In fact, the test is so simple it can even be performed on unborn babies in the womb.

Richard Speck is now behind bars for life, his sentences totaling four hundred years, without a chance of parole. But controversy over the effects of an extra sex chromosome still goes on. After Speck's conviction, one study made in a federal penitentiary indicated that an unusually high number of men on death row carried an extra male chromosome. Another study, though, cast doubt and discredit on these findings. It turned up a number of perfectly law-abiding men who also have two male chromosomes instead of one. Obviously, a long-term study was needed. The results might have far-reaching effects on crime prevention and treatment of certain criminals.

Such a study, implemented by computers, is now in progress at the Medical Center of the University of Massachusetts. Since 1970, researchers have gathered data on the personality traits of a group of children born with three sex chromosomes—either XXY or XYY. Included is a small control group whose chromosome pattern is not typical but who have no extra sex chromosomes.

From birth on, the children have been examined twice a year. They and their parents are interviewed about their habits, hobbies, studies, and friends; how they get along with people; how they see themselves; and how they feel about the opposite sex. All this information is stored in a computer to form a constantly expanding data base. For statistical analysis, the data is relayed by telephone lines to yet another computer at the university's Amherst campus.

The study will not be complete until the youngest child has reached adulthood, sometime around 1990. Most likely, though, the results will banish the idea that people can be driven to crime by their heredity.

HUGE QUANTITIES OF DATA

The Massachusetts study keeps track of only thirty-nine children. Over the years, however, the items of information collected will reach an awe-inspiring number. Other studies deal with data so vast that researchers would have been discouraged from embarking on them before the age of computers. This is especially true of genetic linkage studies, where an attempt is made to follow traits, such as diabetes, hemophilia, or mental retardation in several generations of one family. Following one family's health history back over four generations can generate thousands of items of information.

This is indeed what is happening at the University of California at Los Angeles, where researchers are studying the dermal ridge formation on the hands of autistic children and their parents, in order to link these to other hereditary factors. Autism, a severe disturbance in emotional development, is very rare but sometimes strikes twice in the same family. It may be caused by some biochemical malfunction in the brain, and this, in turn, could have been due to genetic factors. The ridges on the skin of our hands are formed before we are born and never change except in size. The computerized study applies statistical analysis to the total ridge count as well as to the complex shapes of the ridges in an effort to relate these patterns to other developmental characteristics.

One mammoth task that could not possibly have been undertaken without the help of computers is the effort to track down the positions of the human genes, carriers of all hereditary traits. The nuclei of the cells in the human body contain forty-six chromosomes—threadlike structures on which the genes are positioned as subunits. But although chromosomes can be seen under a strong microscope, genes are much too small for observation. The total number of genes determining the heredity of a single human being is estimated to be about three billion. Finding their exact location is a matter of statistical analysis and probability. Only computers can handle such numbers easily. Even so, scientists are still at the beginning of the job. At the present rate of progress, the final solution is centuries away.

EPIDEMIOLOGY

An epidemic is an outbreak of disease affecting many people in one locality. We usually think of epidemics in connection with diseases that spread from person to person, such as chicken pox, or the dreaded ravagers polio, typhus, and cholera. Other diseases can also reach epidemic proportions. Cancer, today, is sometimes thought to be one of them. Finding out where, when, and in what numbers diseases occur leads researchers to discover how they spread and what causes them. Epidemiology—the study of epidemic diseases—is the first step in preventive medicine.

Epidemiology deals with large numbers of cases in diverse geographical regions. Collecting all this information, analyzing it statistically, and storing it as a database for further reference, has been made easier by computers. As a result, more information than ever before is now becoming available on how, when, and where Americans get sick, become well, or die.

New registries—computerized centers for collecting reports on specific illnesses—are formed each year. One of these is a national registry for victims of toxic wastes. Another new registry, kept by the Centers for Disease Control in Atlanta, Georgia, collects facts about patients suffering from the fatal disease AIDS, or Acquired Immune Deficiency Syndrome. AIDS first came to the attention of the American medical community in 1980. By 1983, over fifteen hundred cases had been reported, all but one hundred of them in the United States. The disease, most of whose victims have, until now, been men, seems to be transmitted by sexual contact or by transfusions of blood and blood products.

Scientists are working feverishly to solve the mystery of this illness that has already killed at least one-third of its victims. That is why it is so important to register each new AIDS patient and to study exactly the sort of contact the patient had with other AIDS victims. Telephone wires permit doctors to contact the computer quickly from all parts of the country, either to register or to retrieve data.

MAPPING CANCER MORTALITY

U.S. law mandates that each state collect data on infectious and chronic diseases and on all causes of deaths. Even before this law was passed, several states pioneered the collecting of medical data. Connecticut, for example, founded a tumor registry in 1930, for which it has been gathering valuable information ever since.

When computers came on the scene, such programs became easier to handle and quickly grew in range and scope. The National Center for Health Statistics now has a National Death Registry. This is a central source for other researchers, giving such data as age at death, ethnic background, place of residence, place of death, and cause of death.

A nationwide program now follows all patients who develop cancer. One aim of the program is to estimate chances of survival for patients treated in different ways. Another aim is to find correlations between cancer and life habits, including occupation, alcohol use, smoking, and diet. The cancer registry also uses computers to create geographical maps of cancer incidence and mortality in America. Such computer-generated maps yield surprising discoveries that can help save lives. One map, for instance, reveals a cluster, or unusually high incidence, of mouth and throat cancers among non-white women living in the southeastern United States. This clustering seems to be due to the local custom of snuff dipping, a habit like smoking, that can be avoided for the sake of health.

A BURN REGISTRY

Doctors use large-scale computer-aided studies to help them find ways to prevent or relieve suffering. A registry that has made progress in this direction is the National Burn Information Exchange under the U.S. Public Health Service. The Burn Registry helps to establish the best approach in treating severe burns by comparing methods and results in large numbers of cases. It also reveals important facts, such as that the most frequent burn victims are one- and two-year-olds and that burns are most often received in the kitchen, bathroom, and bedroom.

Most important of all, the registry's figures clearly show that the majority of serious burns are preventable. The most frequent burn accidents happen to children while they are bathing or when they pull pots and pans containing hot liquids off the stove.

One of the first discoveries of the National Burn Information Exchange was that the most devastating injuries occurred when the victim's clothing caught fire. This discovery led to the setting of flammability standards for children's sleepwear and many other fabrics and garments. The findings have been useful in seeking standards for flammability in mattresses and upholstery. Even nonmedical agencies, for example, manufacturers and insurance companies, use the registry to study the probability of fires in places such as boats and tents. These are only some of the ways computers have helped epidemiology expand into the wider fields of preventive medicine and public health.

DRUG RESEARCH WITH COMPUTER GRAPHICS

A research chemist sits in front of a television screen tapping the keys of a computer terminal. On the screen appears a pattern of lines connecting what looks like an array of different colored balls piled next to each other. Strange twisting geometric shapes are displayed, rotated, and moved around to be viewed from all sides.

The balls represent the atoms of the basic building block, the molecule, of a new drug that the scientist is designing. Rather than having to build an awkward wire or ball-and-stick model, or drawing a one-dimensional picture of the drug on paper, the scientist is using a computer to represent the shape of the molecule.

A computer can reproduce molecular shapes far more accurately than can any physical model. Using information stored in data banks on the properties and behavior of atoms, the computer can automatically calculate and display the correct atomic distances, as well as the exact angles between the chemical bonds connecting the atoms. The energy required for different conformations will also be computed so that a correct three-dimensional model of the molecule is produced.

A computer system for graphics that is particularly "friendly," or easy to use, has recently been developed at the University of California. It will accept statements and instructions in basic English rather than in one of the fairly complicated programming languages. Instead of working with a conventional computer terminal, the chemist simply uses a light pen to draw a rough diagram of a particular molecular structure on an electrostatic table. Within seconds, an accurate and stereoscopically correct picture of the molecule appears on a screen. Sitting in front of the screen, the researcher can move and rotate the molecule with two joysticks, as though he or she were playing an electronic game.

DESIGNING DRUGS

Computer graphics are the most recent method of helping to provide people with useful drugs. Using these computer-generated molecules, scientists are able to explore the possible side effects of a new drug by comparing its structure with well-known natural substances. The computer's ability to superimpose and compare the images of several molecules simultaneously permits the scientist to pick out certain arrangements of atoms that are responsible for a particular effect on the body. New drugs can then be designed with the desired atomic arrangement. These may replace the older drugs because they are cheaper and more effective.

Computer graphics were employed by Robert Langridge, director of the Computer Graphics Laboratory at the University of California, to model the way the thyroid hormone thyroxine is bound to the protein that transports it to its target organs. When viewed on the screen, the protein, shown in one color, seemed to contain pockets for holding the iodine atoms of the thyroxine, depicted in another color. It was described jokingly by a fellow scientist: "The binding site of the transport protein is shaped like an olive with the core plugged out, and the hormone fits into that hole like a pimento."

Scientists have used this model to see if they could develop a variation, or "analogue," of the thyroid hormone, one that could be used to improve development in premature infants. It was hoped that the hormone could be administered to the mother before the child was born. Unfortunately, the molecule formed by thyroxine and its protein carrier was too large to pass through the placenta of the pregnant mother. A computer program was then used to design a growth-hormone carrier molecule small enough to reach the unborn baby. Treatment with the hormone has proven successful with rabbits, and there is hope that it will be equally effective with humans.

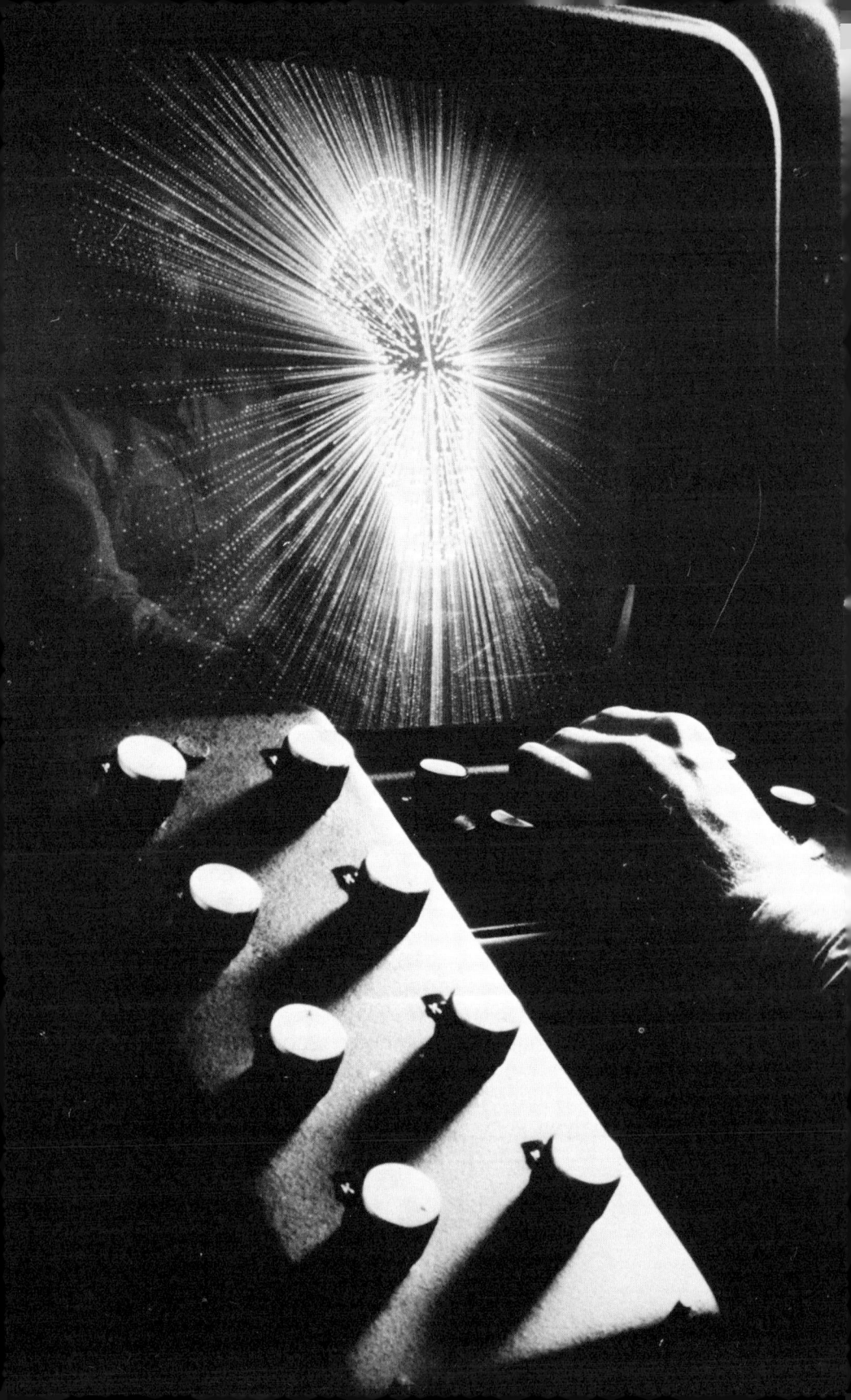

CHEMICAL LOCKS AND KEYS

One of the most successful approaches to the design of drugs assumes that the drug exerts its biological action by interacting with special "receptors" found in the body. The receptor sites may be on a protein molecule bound to a cell membrane, or on an enzyme, or even on the basic molecule of heredity, DNA. Scientists often compare a drug binding to a receptor site to a key fitting a lock. The drug is the "key," which attaches to a receptor "lock." For example, many antibiotics work by fitting into enzyme receptor sites on bacteria and deactivating them. With all the "locks" filled, the enzyme is prevented from functioning normally, and the bacteria dies.

By analyzing and manipulating atomic groups on the molecular models displayed on the screen of a computer, the researcher can tell if a drug's particular arrangement of atoms will serve as a "key" that fits into a particular biological "lock." When the shape of the "key" associated with a drug is unknown, it can often be guessed at by the shape of the receptor-lock it will fit.

Using this technique, researchers at Washington University were able to explain the biological effect of a drug called alloxan. When fed to rats, alloxan produced symptoms usually associated with diabetes. A computer analysis showed that key atomic groups of alloxan resembled

A pharmaceutical researcher works the controls of a three-dimensional computer to manipulate an adenosine molecule, one of the nucleotide bases in DNA.

those of glucose, a sugar molecule that normally causes insulin to be released in the body. They concluded that alloxan fit into the receptor-locks reserved for glucose, inhibiting the release of insulin and inducing the symptoms of diabetes.

Parkinson's disease is associated with the lack of a substance called dopamine, a chemical in the body that aids in transmitting nerve signals. When Professor Garland Marshall of the Washington State School of Medicine wanted to know why four different drugs acted like dopamine, he superimposed all four molecules on a computer to see what, if anything, they contained in common. All the drugs contained the same grouping of carbon and nitrogen atoms at the same location in their structure. The common cluster of atoms was the "key" to the receptors on the nerve endings. This knowlege is expected to be of great value in designing drugs to treat diseases of the nervous system.

Drug design using computer graphics is being used at the New Jersey research laboratories of Merck Sharpe & Dohme. Scientists there are designing and testing a new drug that they hope will help diabetics by controlling the level of sugar in their blood. The compound is a chemical cousin, an "analogue," of somatostatin, a hormone that helps regulate and control blood-sugar levels. The natural hormone itself is ineffective in treating diabetes because it is broken down by the body too quickly to be effective.

Computer analysis of somatostatin showed that only four amino acid groups on the very long and complicated molecule were responsible for the biological activity of the hormone. A team of Merck scientists, led by Daniel F. Veber, then designed a simpler compound, containing the four active groups, that was much more resistant to being broken down. The new compound stays in the body thirty to forty times as long as the natural hormone and shows nearly all the effects of somatostatin in tests on laboratory animals. Dr. Veber stated that "there were so many possible structures that I'm not sure we would have found the correct one without the help of the computer."

ENZYME INHIBITORS

Enzymes are large, complex molecules that control the rate of chemical reactions in the body. A host of diseases, such as high-blood pressure, arthritis, cancer, and heart disease, have been linked to enzyme-induced reactions. The destruction or suppression of the causative enzyme has proven of great value in treating these diseases.

Dr. Douglas Covey, a chemist at the Washington University School of Medicine in St. Louis, has been very active in designing drugs that will destroy enzymes. Using a computer, he models large molecules that resemble the female hormone estrogen and the male hormone testosterone. Their function is to link up with a particular enzyme and inactivate it. Dr. Covey has stated that "molecules could be designed specifically to seek out and kill an enzyme that keeps a tumor growing."

Researchers at Merck have had some success in designing drugs to treat the nonmalignant enlargement of the prostate gland found in aging men. They made use of the fact that special groups of men with unusually small prostates were observed to be missing an enzyme associated with certain male hormones. With the aid of computer graphics they designed a drug that inhibits this enzyme. Although the drug is still in the testing stage, it seems to be a successful inhibitor that shrinks the prostate gland in dogs.

Computer modeling of drugs shows great promise for the future. Cancer and heart disease are only two of the disorders for which new drugs need to be developed. Other computer programs are being developed to try to predict the biological effect of foreign compounds, such as drugs, pesticides, and other toxic chemicals, on the body.

CHAPTER 8

COMPUTERS TO AID THE HANDICAPPED

Although Dave Meltzer was born blind, he came through high school with flying colors. He was quick at learning to read the special print for the blind called braille. Braille consists of raised dots on the page that readers can scan with their fingertips. He also learned touch-typing at an early age.

However, now, as a psychology major in college, Dave cannot find enough braille reading material or recorded cassettes for his needs. Of about 35,000 books published each year, only about one percent is available in braille. An even smaller percentage has been recorded on disks or tape. Dave plans to go on to graduate school, and he needs to read many technical publications as well as books and newspapers.

Each afternoon, Dave slips off to a corner room of the college library. There, he spends a couple of hours in the company of a remarkable computer-aided apparatus

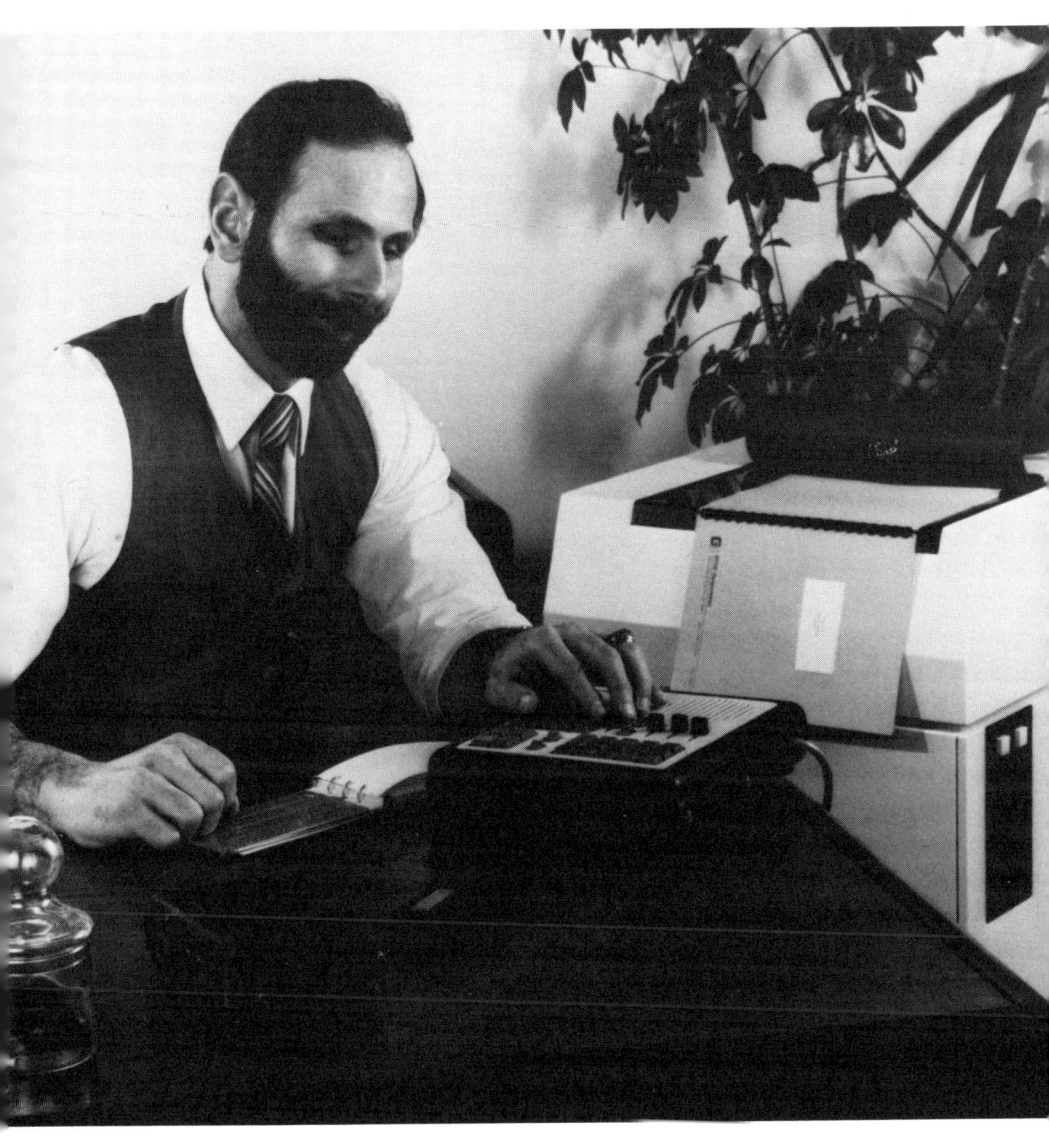

The Kurzweil Reading Machine for the Blind changes printed words into digital signals that are transmitted to a built-in speech synthesizer and read aloud electronically.

called the Kurzweil Reading Machine for the Blind. He places his book or journal on the glass top of the console, which looks very much like a Xerox machine. Then he settles back and listens. A voice begins to read the text. It is rather monotonous because it is a synthetic, electronically produced sound. Its pronunciation is clear, though. Every now and then, when it cannot pronounce an unfamiliar word, it spells it out instead. It reads fairly fast. In fact, it can read up to one-and-a-half times the speed of normal reading.

The Kurzweil reading machine, using optical sensors, can recognize printed characters of almost any shape or size. As the scanner moves across the lines, it converts the images into digital signals and relays these to a microcomputer. The computer uses a unique program that recognizes the letters, groups them into words, and computes the pronunciation of each word.

In its memory, the computer carries over a thousand linguistic rules and fifteen hundred exceptions to these rules. It also carries the rules of English sentence formation, which allow it to give certain words their proper stress. As the computer translates each sentence into electronic impulses, it sends them to a built-in speech synthesizer. The listener can raise or lower the volume and change the speed of the artificial voice.

Because the reading machine can also be programmed to other uses, it has many functions. Blind people can use it as a personal computer and word processor. Through it, they can tune in to a regional information network for the blind. They can also use it to communicate with other blind users in different locations through its audible version of electronic mail.

HELPING PEOPLE TALK

Because Andrew Jay is a victim of severe cerebral palsy, he has little control over his movements and spends his days in a wheelchair. He is an intelligent young man, but his speech is so slurred that he has trouble making himself understood. Recently, though, a California firm called Psycho-Linguistic Research Associates came up with the Versatile, Portable, Speech Prosthesis (VPSP). A prosthesis is any artificial device that substitutes for a part or function of the body. The VPSP has enabled Andrew to speak with the people around him.

The speech prosthesis consists of a microcomputer, a disk drive, a voice synthesizer, a video display, and a speaker. These components are packaged to be as small as possible and are distributed around the wheelchair to keep it in balance and to accommodate the needs of the particular user. Some users can manipulate a keyboard. Others, like Andrew, are not coordinated enough. For them, a different program has been devised that responds to a single switch. The entire system is powered by the batteries of the wheelchair, which are good for a few hours' worth of speech.

To start the system, Andrew flips the switch. The video screen at the side of his wheelchair displays a "menu" of possible choices. A moving dot or cursor proceeds from item to item. To select one of these, Andrew waits until the cursor has moved just above it. Then he touches the switch again. He can select eight cursor speeds, from fast to slow. To speak a pre-stored sentence such as "It's good to see you again" or "Please bring me my sweater," he has only to select the appropriate column, the line he wants to speak, and the talk command. The sentence then issues from the speaker next to his shoulder.

If he wants to compose a phrase, he can choose from a dictionary of nearly one thousand words. He can combine these with a choice of prefixes, endings, connecting words, and possessives. There are also separate pages listing numbers, times of day, places, and a calendar. Picking one's speech with a single switch is slow. But Andrew finds it has made his life better all the same.

HELPING PEOPLE HEAR

As a young girl, Mrs. Propper lost eighty percent of her hearing due to a severe case of typhoid fever. Now, at sixty-five, she is profoundly deaf. All the same, she manages to communicate by means of a typewriterlike instrument called a TDD (Telephone Device for the Deaf), which is connected to her regular telephone. As a resident of California, who has been medically certified as deaf, she receives the equipment free of charge.

The TDD works much like an ordinary telephone. But instead of receiving sound signals, transmitting them as electronic impulses, and changing them back into sound, the TDD receives its signals from a keyboard and conveys them either to a visual display screen or to a printer at the receiving end.

Until recently, though, Mrs. Propper was not entirely comfortable because she could not hear the door or telephone bells. She also worried because she would not be able to hear the smoke alarm in case of fire. Now, she is pleased to have found a computerized wireless system that converts sound signals into flashing lights. The system was installed in her bedroom and sitting room. And now, she can rest easy, knowing that different coded light signals will alert her to several important sounds. She can recognize the doorbell, the telephone, and the smoke alarm.

A computer code that Mrs. Propper can use with her TDD allows her access to a regional electronic mail network for the deaf. This program acts as a news service and bulletin board.

Other devices for the deaf are still in the developing stage. One is a vibrating wristwatch, to be used with a transmitter in one's home. Signals on the watch face could alert deaf wearers to a dozen different sounds, from the ringing of an oven timer to a baby's crying or the barking of the family dog.

KEEPING IN TOUCH

Professor C. V. Brewster was a member of the chemistry department of a midwestern university when he developed a neurological disorder that was soon to leave him physically incapacitated. Professor Brewster knew that he would eventually lose the ability to move his arms and legs, as well as the ability to speak. With great courage and ingenuity, he planned a system of computer-aided devices that would keep him from being entirely helpless. His designs were, in large part, turned into reality by a group of friends and fellow professors at the university.

The system is based on an Apple II computer with a video screen monitor. It is controlled by a single key that the professor can press with his finger. In addition, it is equipped with a floppy disk drive, a printer, a telephone dialer, a light and appliance control device, and a voice synthesizer. These give the invalid a measure of control over his surroundings. From his wheelchair or bed, the professor presses the key and selects from a "menu." He can turn the lights on and off, watch TV, or listen to the radio. He can print out messages. He can telephone a friend by simply picking a number from a list. His telephone set has a microphone-speaker arrangement that bypasses both a receiver and a dial. He speaks by means of the voice synthesizer. In an emergency, he activates a special signal calling for help.

Computerized aids of this kind are valuable in giving people with multiple handicaps some degree of self-determination. What can be done, though, for people so severely disabled that they cannot even press the key that Professor Brewster uses to control his world?

At the Research Institute for Bioengineering in Finland, a switching device was constructed for an eighteen-year-old girl with cerebral palsy. Her condition caused her head and limbs to be in constant involuntary movement. Doctors have found, however, that cerebral palsy patients, even when they have no locomotive power at all, have good control of their lips and tongue. Bioengineers fashioned a device that attached with steel clips behind the young woman's front teeth. It consists of two acrylic plates. When they are brought together, they activate a switch. To give the patient more scope than a mere on-off capacity, therapists at the institute taught her Morse code. The code signals control a computer panel that, in turn, is connected to other appliances. This is how the patient can turn on lights, open and close doors, make a TV selection, and ring an alarm.

Patients unable to move their arms and legs can activate a switch with their chin or with a light spot from a small lamp carried on their forehead. If even this is impossible for them, they can sometimes use a mouthpiece with an air pressure gauge that senses the difference between air being sucked in and blown out. Together with a knowledge of Morse code, such a device empowers severely disabled people to use the microcircuits of a computer for many practical purposes.

SYNTHETIC NERVES

When Carmen Scozzari was seven she felt the first symptoms of a serious disease of the muscle tissues called dystonia musculorum deformans. Within five more years, she had become unable to walk. Eventually, she was forced to spend her days braced and strapped into a wheelchair. Her body was racked by constant muscle spasms.

At twenty-nine, Carmen was referred to Dr. Joseph M. Waltz of St. Barnabas Hospital in the Bronx, New York. Dr. Waltz was known for his treatment of disorders of the nervous system by electrical stimulation of the spinal cord. He operated on Carmen Scozzari by implanting four tiny platinum electrodes high in her spinal cord near the neck. Fine steel wires connect the electrodes to a receiver inserted under the skin in her side. A microprocessor gives off electrical impulses that are picked up by the receiver, activating the wires to stimulate the spinal cord.

The microprocessor, which is no larger than a wallet, hangs on the patient's belt. It has a control panel for selecting the intensity and frequency of the signals and any combination of settings. After a few weeks of learning to tune the microprocessor, Carmen was able to walk without help. She has discarded her arm and leg braces and is free of pain.

NEUROPROTHESIS FOR THE BLIND

The electrodes and microprocessor that enable Carmen to walk act as a synthetic nervous system. Any device that replaces non-functioning nerves is called a neuroprosthesis. Neuroprostheses for the blind are now in the experimental stage. In normal seeing, light and color from the outside world enter the eye and stimulate the cells of the retina at the back of the eyeball. As a result of this stimulation, the cells send electrical impulses to the visual cortex—the area of the brain concerned with vision. This is the part that interprets the impulses that reach it, the part that tells us what we are seeing.

When the eyes are blind, some other instrument must be found to receive outside impulses. By implanting numerous electrodes in the patient's visual cortex, outside impulses can be captured. Each time an electrode is stimulated, it produces a perception of a spot of light somewhere in the patient's visual field.

In one prosthetic device, a tiny radio receiver and an electronic logic circuit are enclosed in a skull cap worn over the patient's head. A thin cable enters the skull through an opening above the back of the neck and runs to the array of cortical electrodes. When the electrodes are stimulated in a regular pattern, the patient receives a perception of shapes. This little computerized device is expected, someday, to enable blind people to read printed lettering and see simple outlines.

Dr. P. E. K. Donaldson of Great Britain built his first vision prosthesis with eighty electrodes but has now increased this number to two hundred. In the future, he projects inserting some eight hundred implants. He believes this will allow patients to "see" in far greater detail.

ARTIFICIAL JOINT IMPLANTS

Nick Tyson went to college on a football scholarship. Early in his career, he injured his left knee but disregarded the pain and continued to play. Later in the season, he hurt the same knee twice more. Each time, he shrugged off the injury. By the time Nick reached his senior year, he was forced to give up football. The knee joint had grown so stiff that he could no longer bend his left leg.

Nick consulted an orthopedic surgeon who decided the best solution would be to replace the injured knee joint with an artificial implant. Other specialists agreed.

Joint replacement surgery is a relatively recent development in medicine. Because it is a highly successful procedure, it has gained widespread acceptance. Knees and hips are the joints most often replaced, but the operation can also be performed on elbows, shoulders, and finger joints. Joint replacement can benefit accident victims and bone-cancer patients. Chiefly, though, it benefits elderly people whose joints have become deformed, stiff, and painful due to arthritis.

Until recently, the artificial joint to be implanted had to be made entirely by hand. First, the surgeon worked with a bioengineer to create a specific design. Then, a highly skilled machinist spent many hours cutting and shaping the device out of titanium—the metal most commonly used for the job. Even so, many adjustments in the fit of the implant to the patient's own bone structure had to be made on the operating table.

Today, the use of computers has made the preparation of implants more accurate, faster, and less expensive. In 1976, surgeons and bioengineers at the Hospital for Special Surgery in New York City joined efforts with some of the faculty at Cornell's School of Mechanical and Aerospace Engineering. Together, they developed a three-stage, computer-assisted system that can select, design, and manufacture artificial knee and hip joints. (Computer design of other joints is expected to follow soon.) The system is called CAPS/CAD/CAM, which is short for Computer-Assisted Prosthesis Selection/Computer-Assisted Design/Computer-Assisted Manufacture.

The first stage of the process uses CT (Computerized Tomography) scanning to obtain three-dimensional images of the patient's joint structure. (For more about CT scanning, see the chapter in this book on body imaging.) The patient's age, height, weight, and physical condition are also added to the computer's store of information.

Using all the data, the computer scans through the standard designs programmed into its memory to select the one that most closely matches the particular patient's needs. If the surgeon examining the selected model does not find it entirely suitable, however, he or she can use the system to prepare a custom-designed implant.

Sitting in front of the terminal, the surgeon is able to view the patient's bone image and to manipulate it almost as in actual surgery. Because the computer needs added information to change or modify a design, it has been programmed to ask the surgeon a number of questions. The process of selecting even a complicated custom-designed implant takes no longer than ten minutes.

As soon as the surgeon is satisfied with the model of the implant, the computer creates a blueprint for the

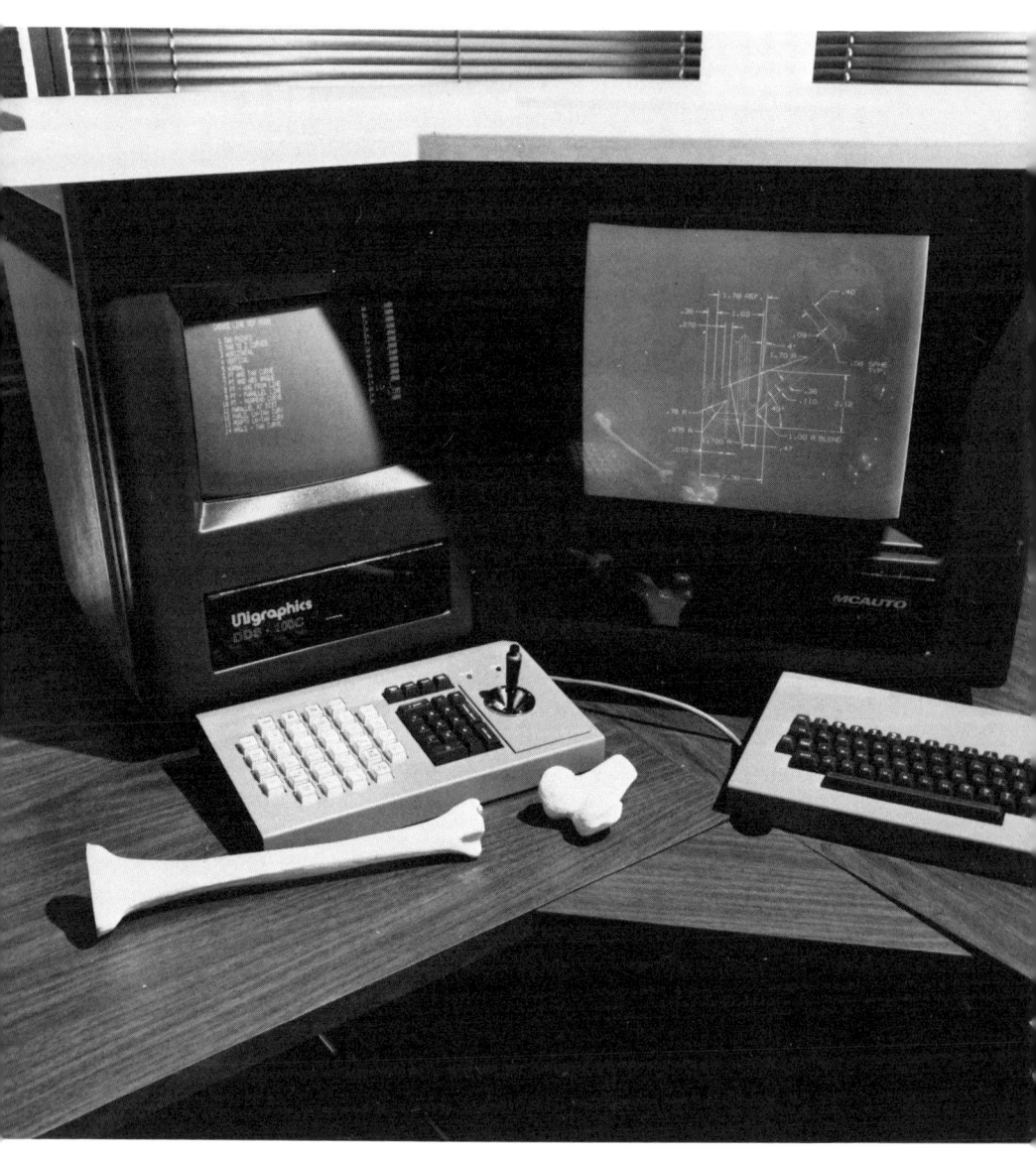

The CAPS/CAD/CAM system in use at the Hospital for Special Surgery in New York City selects, designs, and manufactures artificial knee and hip joints.

manufacturing process. It punches out coded instructions on paper tape, giving precise directions to the machines that will cut and shape the artificial joint.

The lathes and milling machines involved in the last part of the process are astoundingly precise and fast. They cut metal to within 1/10,000 of an inch, following computer-designed instructions to round an edge or curve a certain line. The entire job, formerly so time-consuming, is finished in a little more than an hour. Only polishing and sterilizing are needed now, and the device is ready for the patient.

Most patients are delighted with the results of knee or hip replacement. They can once again walk without stiffness and are completely relieved of pain.

FUTURE DEVELOPMENTS

Another device to help the disabled is still in the works. This one is the exact reverse of the Kurzweil reading machine. Instead of turning print into speech, it proposes to turn speech into print. Its sound-sensors are expected to interface with a computer to digitize the spoken word. The data would be converted to letters displayed on a screen or on a printer. Just as the voice synthesizer is of value to the blind, a print synthesizer would be of service to the deaf.

Perhaps one day, we will have computer-aided home environments to allow very elderly people to live comfortably alone. Imagine an aged man who is sound in limb but failing in memory. A system could be engineered around him to remind him of important things to do, such as turning off the stove or taking along the housekeys before shutting the front door. A pleasant synthetic voice could tell him that it's time to take his medication: "One of the large blue pills and two of the small white ones and don't forget to drink a full glass of water afterwards." Around dinnertime it could remind him that his sister left two portions of stuffed peppers in the freezer for him on a recent visit.

The system's sensors might even be geared to detect something wrong if the old gentleman stayed in bed past his usual time for rising. "Are you feeling all right this morning?" the system could be programmed to ask. Then, if it received no answer, it could turn in an alarm to a relative or to some designated emergency service.

These are only a few of the ways in which computers can be applied to the needs of the disabled. The field of computerized medicine is new, and each year of the past decade has brought tremendous innovations. No doubt, this trend will continue for some time to come. For those who hope to make their career in some area of computer-aided medicine, there is great work ahead.

INDEX

Accuracy controls, 53
Acquired Immune Deficiency Syndrome (AIDS), 67-68
Admissions, hospital, 13
Artificial joints, 84-87
Autism, 66
Auxiliary systems, 25

Billing, hospital, 21
Bits and bytes, 23-24
Blind, the, 76-78, 83, 87
Blood chemistry, 48
Blood gas, 49
Body imaging, 30-46
Burn registry, 69

Cancer, 67, 68-69
CAPS/CAD/CAM, 85
Cardiac output, measuring, 60-62
Cardiogenic shock, 56-57
Central computer, 20-29

Central processing unit (CPU), 21-22
Cerebral palsy, 81-82
Chemical locks and keys, 73-75
Chromosome defects, 64-65
Computed tomography (CT), 7-8, 30-33, 42, 85
Confidentiality, 17-18
Console terminal, 22

Data bases, 27-28
Deaf, the, 80, 87
Diagnosis, 4-5, 30-55
Digital subtraction angiography, 34-36
Drug research and design, 70-75

Electrocardiogram (ECG), 57-60
Electroencephalogram (EEG), 53
Enzyme inhibitors, 75
Epidemiology, 67-68
Evoked potentials, 53-55

Extended Binary Coded Interchange Code (EBCDIC), 23

Fees, hospital, 17

Genetic testing, 64–67
Graphics, computer, 8–9, 70, 71, 74

Handicapped, computer aid for, 76–88
Heart disease, 38, 39–40, 58
Hematrak, 52
Hospital systems, 10–19

Intensive care, 56–63
Interview, computer, 1–3

Joints, artificial, 84–87

Magnetic disk, 26–27
Magnetic tape, 25–26
Modems, 24–25

Nerves, synthetic, 82–83
Network control, 24
Neuroprothesis, 83–84
Non-invasive tests, 55
Nuclear magnetic resonance (NMR), 40–41

Organ registry, 5–7

Positron emission tomography (PET), 42–46

Radiation therapy, 38–39
Radiology, 47–48
Repairs, 29
Research, 64–75

Safeguarding system, 28–29
Safety, patient, 18–19
Sequential Multiple Analyzer Computer (SMAC), 49–51
Speech prothesis, 79
Surgery, 7–9, 84–85
Synthetic nerves, 82–83

Telemetry, 63
Telephone Device for the Deaf (TDD), 80
Tissue-typing, 6–7
Transplants, 5–7

Ultrasonography, 36–38

Vital signs, 60–63

X rays, 31–36, 39, 48